101 Questions to Ask Y...

Dr Tom Smith has been writing since 1977, after spending six years in general practice and seven years in medical research. He writes the 'Doctor, Doctor' column in *The Guardian* on Saturdays, and has written three humorous books, *Doctor, Have You Got a Minute?*, *A Seaside Practice* and *Going Loco*, all published by Short Books. His other books for Sheldon Press include *Heart Attacks: Prevent and Survive*, *Living with Alzheimer's Disease*, *Overcoming Back Pain*, *Coping with Bowel Cancer*, *Coping with Heartburn and Reflux*, *Coping with Age-related Memory Loss*, *Skin Cancer: Prevent and Survive*, *How to Get the Best from Your Doctor*, *Coping with Kidney Disease*, *Osteoporosis: Prevent and Treat* and *Coping Successfully with Prostate Cancer*.

A L I S

3047299

Overcoming Common Problems Series

Selected titles

A full list of titles is available from Sheldon Press,
36 Causton Street, London SW1P 4ST and on our website at
www.sheldonpress.co.uk

101 Questions to Ask Your Doctor
Dr Tom Smith

Asperger Syndrome in Adults
Dr Ruth Searle

The Assertiveness Handbook
Mary Hartley

Assertiveness: Step by step
Dr Windy Dryden and Daniel Constantinou

Backache: What you need to know
Dr David Delvin

Body Language: What you need to know
David Cohen

Bulimia, Binge-eating and their Treatment
Professor J. Hubert Lacey, Dr Bryony Bamford and
Amy Brown

The Cancer Survivor's Handbook
Dr Terry Priestman

The Chronic Pain Diet Book
Neville Shone

Cider Vinegar
Margaret Hills

Coeliac Disease: What you need to know
Alex Gazzola

Confidence Works
Gladeana McMahon

Coping Successfully with Pain
Neville Shone

Coping Successfully with Prostate Cancer
Dr Tom Smith

Coping Successfully with Psoriasis
Christine Craggs-Hinton

Coping Successfully with Ulcerative Colitis
Peter Cartwright

Coping Successfully with Varicose Veins
Christine Craggs-Hinton

Coping Successfully with Your Hiatus Hernia
Dr Tom Smith

Coping Successfully with Your Irritable Bowel
Rosemary Nicol

Coping When Your Child Has Cerebral Palsy
Jill Eckersley

Coping with Age-related Memory Loss
Dr Tom Smith

Coping with Birth Trauma and Postnatal Depression
Lucy Jolin

Coping with Bowel Cancer
Dr Tom Smith

Coping with Bronchitis and Emphysema
Dr Tom Smith

Coping with Candida
Shirley Trickett

Coping with Chemotherapy
Dr Terry Priestman

Coping with Chronic Fatigue
Trudie Chalder

Coping with Coeliac Disease
Karen Brody

Coping with Compulsive Eating
Dr Ruth Searle

Coping with Diabetes in Childhood and Adolescence
Dr Philippa Kaye

Coping with Diverticulitis
Peter Cartwright

Coping with Dyspraxia
Jill Eckersley

Coping with Early-onset Dementia
Jill Eckersley

Coping with Eating Disorders and Body Image
Christine Craggs-Hinton

Coping with Envy
Dr Windy Dryden

Coping with Epilepsy in Children and Young People
Susan Elliot-Wright

Coping with Family Stress
Dr Peter Cheevers

Coping with Gout
Christine Craggs-Hinton

Coping with Hay Fever
Christine Craggs-Hinton

Coping with Headaches and Migraine
Alison Frith

Coping with Hearing Loss
Christine Craggs-Hinton

Overcoming Common Problems Series

Overcoming Common Problems Series

101 Questions to Ask Your Doctor

DR TOM SMITH

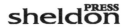

First published in Great Britain in 2011

Sheldon Press
36 Causton Street
London SW1P 4ST
www.sheldonpress.co.uk

The author and publisher have made every effort to ensure that the
external website and email addresses included in this book are correct and
up to date at the time of going to press. The author and publisher are not
responsible for the content, quality or continuing accessibility of the sites.

British Library Cataloguing-in-Publication Data
A catalogue record for this book is available from the British Library

ISBN 978-1-84709-145-1

1 3 5 7 9 10 8 6 4 2

Typeset by Fakenham Prepress Solution, Fakenham, Norfolk NR21 8NN
Printed in Great Britain by Ashford Colour Press

Produced on paper from sustainable forests

For Mary

Contents

Introduction

One of the abiding memories of my boyhood was a picture on my grandfather's wall. Called 'The Doctor', it showed a distinguished man with a grey beard sitting by the bed of a sick girl. He is full of deep thought, looking into the distance. The child is ashen-faced, lying semi-conscious, dying.

Luke Fildes' painting was a favourite of the Victorians, reminding them of the reverence in which they held their doctors and of the fragility of life. The doctor–patient relationship was a one-way process: knowledge and wisdom flowed from doctor to patient, and the family was properly in awe of him. In those times the doctor was, of course, always male.

Something of that reverence remained into the last half of the twentieth century. As a young doctor in hospital and in my early years in practice I was acutely aware of the expectations my patients had of me, and that it was almost impossible to live up to them. If the patients put us on a pedestal, we were well warned by our teachers not to climb on to it ourselves.

Even as a small boy, I knew that my grandfather took a very different view of the painting from me. He was attracted by the patrician figure of the doctor, and I was saddened by the figure on the bed. For me the doctor was irrelevant. Why was he not doing something to cure the child, instead of simply waiting for her to die? My Victorian grandparents loved that doctor – I saw him as a hopeless irrelevance. He had a wonderful bedside manner, but it was of absolutely no help to the child. What he needed was something to cure her illness – and in Victorian times he didn't have it.

Whenever I hear that a doctor has 'a great bedside manner' I think of that painting. Maybe I have it, maybe I don't. But what we do have, these days, is the ability to cure so many people of their illnesses, and that takes precedence.

Medicine has changed generally. The old emotional 'feel' between doctor and patient has diminished, and in doing so it has altered fundamentally the old relationship between us. We have become scientists with a specific job to do for each person we see, and you have had to become content with much less of our time. Communications between us have had to become concise and effective for your illnesses to be understood, diagnosed and treated, and the bedside manner is much less relevant.

The positive side of this sad (I as a doctor feel the sadness as much as you do as a patient) change is that we are far more able, in every sphere of medicine, to offer you treatments that really work and will not only make you feel better, but also keep you from serious harm. It starts with the way we are all trained in medical school. We are taught how to talk to patients, how to take a history, to perform the appropriate examinations and tests, to come to a diagnosis, then initiate treatment or refer to a specialist. It explains how the consultation isn't random, but highly structured, so as to be efficient and also fast and accurate. It also explains how patients, seeing their doctors for the first time, can help or hinder them in the process. As each consultation is scheduled to take around ten minutes, that's vital.

You may find you have quite different perceptions from your doctor's about what the initial consultation is about and how it should proceed. You may also be surprised about the need for follow-up, and how you and your doctor will develop a long-term relationship around your illness. We spend much more time than we used to on following up illnesses or preventing potential illnesses, and there are plenty of examples, taken from my own experience as a doctor, for you to compare with your own experiences.

This book covers some of the topics that tend to get left out of this process. Today's tailored consultations don't always leave room for the random, the quirky and the plain trivial. That's where these questions come in. As you'll see, they're quite a mixture, from general medical knowledge, to questions that are so specialized that only one person may ever have asked them.

One point I would like to make: they are all genuine. That is, every question has really been asked by a real person at some point. Some of them have come to me via the pages of *The Guardian*, where I've been doing my best to answer such queries for a number of years. Others may have been put to me at parties in more or less unguarded moments. Still others may be the 'hand on the doorknob' or the 'while I'm here' variety, that get popped out just as the patient is leaving the surgery after a consultation ostensibly about something else. For this reason, they may echo very real fears the person may have, too. But I hope that, for whatever reason you're reading this book, you'll find the answers reassuring and informative. And if you need to know more, or are seriously worried about something, do visit your own GP and ask your own questions.

1

Obesity

Q: I've read that there are two different types of obesity – apples, who put weight on around the middle, and pears, who put it on round the hips. The article stated that the 'apples' are at higher risk than 'pears' of heart attacks. Is there any statistical basis for this? Do you have figures for how high the risk is for a given waist measurement? I'm an apple, by the way.

A: Waist circumference is a good guide to the risk of early death. In a study of nearly 400,000 healthy Europeans, each added 5 cm of waist measurement increased men's risk of early death by 17 per cent and the women's risk by 13 per cent. Interestingly the link was higher if the person had a relatively low body mass index – so that if you have a paunch, but are not very muscular, you are at the highest risk. That's confirmed by another study concluding that a thicker calf muscle in old age may protect you against heart attacks. A high waist-to-hip ratio (more fat around the waist than hips) also indicates a higher than normal risk. So apples should really try to shed the abdominal fat. Sorry.

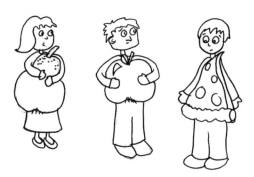

Q: My 12-year-old son and I are both overweight and want to choose an exercise to help us lose the excess. We have tried swimming up and down a pool and find it boring, so we are thinking of jogging or cycling. What are their advantages and disadvantages?

A: The big advantage of cycling for you is that the saddle takes 70 per cent of your body weight, sparing your hip joints while your muscles improve and you shed your excess fat. In jogging your hip and knee joints have to cope with forces between two and three times your body weight. That's a huge strain until you get nearer to a normal body shape. So cycling has the advantage, initially, over running. However, much depends on how much you enjoy either activity, and whether or not you can both cycle in safety. You need less kit when running, except that when running on roads and pavements you must have shoes that absorb the shock of pounding on them. Can you cycle to work and school? That would be a good start, and would help your son's self-confidence, too.

Q: I have put on five stones since I married ten years ago. Diets don't work. What else can I do?

A: Losing weight is never just about eating less. You must also exercise more. If you keep eating a variety of food while cutting down on the amount and never rushing a meal, and add a brisk hour's walk every day, you are bound to lose weight. You will feel fitter, be ready for more exercise, and your appetite will lessen, too. You will then be in a virtuous circle of losing weight, rather than a vicious circle of gaining. When eating, reduce the amount you usually put on your fork or spoon, chew it more slowly, and put down the cutlery between bites. Take at least 20 minutes over your main course, so that your 'anti-hunger' chemistry kicks in before you have finished your meal. Then you will find you have eaten less at each meal, without making you ravenous. Drinking plenty of water with each meal helps too.

Q: Is it true that for some people becoming fat is a matter of a different metabolism from normal, and not because they eat too much or exercise too little?

A: No, it's not. The human metabolic rate, that is the rate at which we burn foods to provide us with energy, is very strictly controlled, and varies very little from one person to another. Think about your body temperature. Everyone knows that it is 37 degrees Celsius, and the slightest increase or decrease in it denotes some form of illness – like a fever or hypothermia. The body's metabolism in normal health is geared to work within very strict limits and at this very controlled temperature. The metabolic rate only alters in illness or under conditions of real stress.

One example comes from problems with the thyroid gland. It helps regulate our metabolic rate. If it is overactive, we do every-thing faster, at a higher heart rate. We are physically overactive and have a ravenous appetite, but lose weight. If it is under-active, everything slows down, including our heart rate and our mental processes, and we put on weight. Both these conditions are illnesses, and if your thyroid gland is normal your obesity can't be laid at its door.

For stress to change your metabolism, you need to be under attack by a sabre-tooth cat (the old hunter-gatherer example) or by your average high street mugger. Or perhaps you are watching, on TV, world politicians making a mess of things again. The urge to fight, or to flee from, an enemy will release a surge of adrenalin that will increase your metabolism for a while. However, that is just temporary, and your metabolism soon returns to normal when the threat has passed. Unless you are in a state of constant anger or fear for every waking hour, which is in effect an illness, your metabolism will remain inside the strict limits set for every human being, in the same way as your temperature does.

Q: My friend has brought back from America some ma huang. She says it helps her lose weight. What is your opinion on it?
A: You should not use it. Its other name is ephedra, and it contains a lot of chemicals that stimulate the heart, one of which is the prescription drug ephedrine. It is on the banned list for athletes. Ma huang side effects are reported to be much worse than those from ginkgo biloba and kava, two other popular alternative herbal remedies. Among them are a very fast heart rate and a rise in blood pressure. Don't be fooled into thinking that because it's 'natural' it can't be dangerous. Deadly nightshade, foxglove and monkshood are natural, but you wouldn't dream of taking them.

Q: What is it that makes me so hungry all the time? I'm sure that it's what has made me fat.
A: Whether we are hungry or not depends on the levels of a substance called leptin in our blood. Leptin is released by fat cells into the circulation after we have started to eat a substantial meal. When it reaches the brain, it attaches to nerve cells in the 'hunger centre' deep in the brain. That switches off our feeling of hunger, and we stop eating.

So why don't we use leptin to lose weight? Shouldn't we take a dose of it, switch off our hunger mechanisms, and slice off the pounds? Sadly, it doesn't work as simply as that. Overweight people actually produce a lot of leptin naturally, but they also produce a protein called CRP in fairly large quantities. CRP destroys the circulating leptin before it has a chance to bind to the hunger cells, so they don't switch off their hunger. The more leptin we give to an obese person, the more CRP they produce, so that giving leptin will never be the answer for them. It seems that what we need to do is to find a way of shutting down CRP production. The scientists are working on it, but don't hold your breath – it may just introduce other complications into the hunger–satiety balance.

2

Diabetes

Q: I have diabetes and have had minor heart problems: I have had chest pains on doing fairly strenuous exercise. My doctor advised me to take aspirin every day to prevent a heart attack or stroke, but a recent press report suggested that it doesn't work. Do I really have to take it?

A: The report (on 2,500 Japanese adults) was on the taking of aspirin to prevent complications in people with diabetes who are otherwise healthy. They had so few trial 'events' (illnesses) that it was impossible to show whether or not aspirin helped or worsened their prospects of heart and circulation complications. (Diabetes raises the risk of both.) As you already have a heart problem, that trial was irrelevant to you: your doctor is following standard guidelines in prescribing aspirin. Whether it will help to prevent heart attacks and strokes in diabetes without any sign, yet, of vascular complications, was the subject of two large trials. They both suggested that aspirin would help prevent circulation problems in diabetics of either type (insulin and non-insulin dependent), so GPs like myself routinely prescribe it for them, unless there is a direct contra-indication (such as a previous reaction to aspirin, stomach ulcers or inflammation, or bleeding problems).

Q: I have diabetes, and my doctor has asked me to take a statin drug daily to lower my cholesterol, along with an aspirin and drugs to lower my blood pressure, over and above my usual diabetes tablets. Why do I have to take so many medicines, especially as my blood pressure and my cholesterol levels aren't all that high?

A: Your big risk, as a type 2 diabetic, is not actually your diabetes, but your higher than average chances of a heart attack or stroke. That's because in diabetes your arteries are particularly prone to fatty degeneration and to damage from high blood pressure. There's good evidence that keeping both the cholesterol and the blood pressure at the lower end of the normal range helps prevent a substantial number of heart attacks and strokes, especially in people with diabetes. They also prevent blindness, kidney failure and circulation problems in your legs. Statins and blood pressure lowering drugs are the best way (along with a healthy lifestyle) of achieving those aims. The aspirin helps to prevent clots forming in your arteries – yet another risk in diabetes. So you are enjoying the best of modern treatment for your diabetes.

Q: My brother-in-law has just been diagnosed as having diabetes, and has to use insulin. He is still driving. What are the rules about this? Isn't it dangerous for him to drive?

A: He must tell the DVLA (Driving and Vehicle Licensing Agency) about his illness: he is breaking the law if he doesn't. He will be sent the new rules when he does, in a leaflet. Put simply, he should test for blood glucose before driving, and if it is below 4 mmol/litre he shouldn't drive. He should first eat, then wait for 45 minutes after it has risen above 5 mmol/litre before setting off. He should take his glucose meter with him in the car, test every two hours, and stop and snack if the glucose level drops below 5. These are not just arbitrary rules that can be bent. He should strictly observe them, as a dropping blood glucose level greatly reduces his ability to drive, slowing reaction times and increasing errors of judgement, greatly increasing his chances of causing an accident.

Q: I've been recently diagnosed as a type 2 diabetic. I'm exercising more, eating wisely, and have stopped smoking, but how can I get rid of my sweet tooth? I have a very difficult time passing a sweet shop.

A: Stop eating sugary foods, including sugar in tea and coffee. Absolutely *don't* drink 'diet' drinks with sweeteners in them, because they will keep your craving for sweet things going. Don't take sweeteners in your tea or coffee, for the same reason. Instead, start to enjoy savoury foods. Indulge in fresh fruit because the sugar in fruit takes longer to digest than refined sugars, and that's important in lessening your need to produce insulin. After about a month you will realize that you are tasting food better, and you don't really need sweetness. When someone puts sugar in your coffee you could well be revolted by it. Hard to believe? Millions of people in your position have managed the transition successfully.

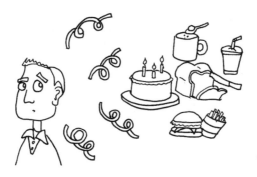

Q: I have diabetes and angina, but my real worry is pain in my feet and hands. It is worst at night. Painkillers don't help, and it is making me miserable. Would manipulation help?

A: I advise very strongly against manipulation as this sounds much more like neuropathy – an inflammation of the nerves in the limbs that can complicate diabetes. Manipulation may make it even worse. Instead discuss it with your diabetes specialist: your best answer may be to take better control over your diabetes. Normal painkillers don't help this type of pain, but it may respond to antidepressant drugs, or to drugs that were initially designed for epilepsy, which 'damp down' the abnormal impulses in nerves affected by neuropathy. Your doctor will advise.

Q: My husband has had diabetes insipidus since an aneurysm burst in his brain. Could you explain this?

A: The aneurysm (which is like a small balloon on a blood vessel) must have damaged his pituitary gland (which is in the middle of the head) when it burst. One of the actions of the pituitary is to control the amount of fluid excreted by the kidneys, by secreting into the bloodstream a substance called anti-diuretic hormone (ADH). Without ADH the kidneys excrete very much more urine than usual. Diabetes insipidus is the name of this condition, in which people produce literally gallons of urine a day and have to drink extra fluids to keep up with the outflow. Happily we can give an ADH equivalent, desmopressin, either by injection or as a spray into the nose, to correct the problem.

3

The heart and high blood pressure

Q: For more than a year I've been getting pains in my left armpit, my left arm and into my jaw. It isn't in my chest. My doctor says it may be my heart. How is that possible, if I don't have chest pain?

A: Any left-sided pain in shoulder, face and arm must be considered as coming from the heart unless proven otherwise by tests. Your doctor will want to know the type of pain (dull and aching, or sharp and burning) and when it comes on (with exercise or after food), and what eases it (rest or antacids). The answers will shed light on whether the pain is from your heart or elsewhere.

Q: Is garlic really good for the heart, and if so why?

A: It depends on what sort of heart problem you think you may develop. If you fear a clot in your coronary arteries – a coronary thrombosis – then enzymes in garlic (thiosulphinate and allicin) help prevent clots forming. However, cooking garlic for more than five minutes destroys them. You have to crush it first (to break down cell walls) to make the enzymes available for digestion. So eat nearly raw crushed garlic to get the best out of it. On the downside, if you bleed too easily, or if you are taking a prescribed anticoagulant, say warfarin, crushed raw garlic may make things worse. It's a matter of balance between clotting and bleeding. As for the claim that garlic lowers cholesterol levels, recent studies refute it. Why not just enjoy garlic as a tasty food, and not look on it as a medicine?

Q: My dentist says that my plaque build-up is due to age-related blood chemistry changes. I'm 68. How may these changes affect

9

my cardiovascular health? My mother and her three siblings all developed vascular dementia in their eighties.

A: I'm no dentist, but my medical information on plaque is that it depends mostly on the bacteria within the mouth, the volume and pH (acidity/alkalinity) of saliva, and how well you have cared for your teeth and gums. There is an easy way to answer your question: see your doctor, who will take a blood test to check your biochemistry. At 68 you are due for a review, anyway, of your kidney, liver and cardiovascular functions, and all these would reflect your cardiovascular health more accurately than your dental plaque.

I don't know of research relating vascular dementia to dental plaque. The main correlates for cardiovascular risk are with untreated high blood pressure, smoking, high cholesterol, poorly controlled diabetes, obesity and lack of regular aerobic exercise. Your mother and her three siblings may well have differed from you in all of these: you cannot relate your own risk to theirs.

Q: I had a heart attack three months ago, and frankly I'm fairly depressed about it. I always thought I was invincible: now I'm facing my own mortality for the first time. How can I resolve this?

A: You are not alone. One in five post-heart attack patients develops major depression within weeks, and another quarter is moderately depressed. If you remain depressed your risk of another attack rises slightly, so do seek professional help. Happily, you will have plenty of support from your rehabilitation team. The British Heart Foundation runs a stress management course (using a publication called *The Heart Manual*) that works well and has been proven to lighten depression. Ask your doctor about it. Follow the advice given: in your depressed state you may not feel like bothering. The closer you comply with both your antidepressant drugs and non-drug treatment the better you will feel, and the faster you will recover.

Q: What does a pacemaker do? My husband has been told he needs one.

A: It controls the rate at which the heart beats. So if your husband's heartbeat is too slow or too fast, it will make it beat at the right speed for him. If he is having runs of abnormal beats, the pacemaker can stop those, too. He should feel a lot easier and fitter with the pacemaker.

Q: My consultant tells me that I have a sinus bradycardia with first degree block. What does this mean? Could it be the result of a heart attack, and would I benefit from heart surgery?

A: It means that your heart is beating slower than normal, and that the beat is not passing normally from the upper chambers of your heart (your 'atria') to your lower chambers (your 'ventricles'). This could have been caused by your heart attack. As for heart surgery, whether you might benefit will depend on a whole series of tests to see if the way your heart beats can be altered. You may need a pacemaker, rather than surgery.

Q: I've just been put on amiodarone tablets to correct an abnormal heart rhythm. I'm told I have to avoid sitting in the sun. Is this really true? I love sunshine holidays.

A: Please keep in the shade. Amiodarone can make you very sensitive to sunlight, giving rashes and a mauve appearance, especially in the cheeks.

Q: I have a 'flabby heart' due to a leaking valve. What advice can you give?

A: I'm not sure what you mean by a flabby heart. Usually the heart muscle grows thicker and stronger if a valve is leaking, because it has to cope with the extra work it has to do. Has your doctor discussed heart valve replacement surgery with you? It sounds as if this has to be one of your options. If you actually have heart failure, then there are modern treatments for that, too.

Q: I am Muslim and have heart disease, so I'm on medicines for high blood pressure and angina. What should I do in Ramadan? Can I fast during the day?

A: I don't know why not. Fasting during the day may even be beneficial for you. Cholesterol levels fall in men fasting for Ramadan, so reducing your chances of a heart attack or stroke. You should still discuss the benefits and drawbacks of fasting with your doctor, but on the whole it shouldn't cause problems for you. Non-Muslims might well benefit from following Ramadan.

Q: I take warfarin to stop clots forming on a new heart valve. I've also been taking cranberry juice for cystitis, but my doctor says they are not compatible. Why is this, and what should I take instead for my urinary infections?

A: Your doctor is correct. Cranberry juice may increase the effect of the clot-preventing drug so that you may start to bleed. If you are taking cranberry juice you need more frequent blood tests to check on your clotting times. Drinking plain water instead may be better for you. If you are having frequent urine infections, take samples to your doctor for culture to find the cause and the appropriate antibiotic to use against it.

Q: Heart attacks run in our family – my father and two uncles died from them, and I think my grandfather may have had one, too. What are my risks of having one? I'm male, 55, slim, don't smoke and have a normal blood pressure. My brother says heart attacks are more a matter of lifestyle and not inheritance – and we live very differently from the previous generation. He says I shouldn't worry.

A: Much depends on the age at which your relatives had their heart attacks. If they were men under 55 years old (or women under 65 years old), then you may be at more risk than most, regardless of your lifestyle. If that's the case in your family, then ask your doctor to assess your risk. That can be done from your previous medical history, your blood pressure, smoking and drinking habits, your body mass index (a measure of how fat you are) and your cholesterol levels. You may be asked to have an exercise ECG if there are any signs of heart disease. And you may be asked to take an aspirin a day – that has been proved to reduce heart attack risk in people especially susceptible to coronary heart disease.

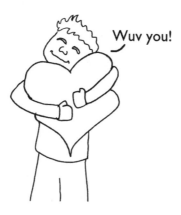

Q: Last September it was confirmed that I have an abdominal aortic aneurysm. This week an ECG indicated a problem with my left ventricle. How common are these two conditions together? Can the aneurysm mimic a ventricle problem? I am male, 69, and in reasonably good health.

A: The two often go together as they are the consequence of the same problem. It's called atherosclerosis, and is caused by fatty degeneration in the lining of the arteries and the heart. It is usually the end product of years of the combination of high circulating cholesterol in the blood, high blood pressure and damage due to smoking (the combination itself of carbon monoxide, nicotine and many different tars, all of which damage the lining cells of the arteries). Your doctor will want to control the pressure, to bring down the fat levels (probably with a statin drug), to know that you have smoked your last cigarette, and to monitor the size of the aneurysm, so that if it enlarges further you can be referred for surgery.

Q: Is it true that people today have fewer heart attacks than a generation ago? How does this fit with the fact that far more people are obese now than then?
A: Yes, it's true. There has been a massive 60 per cent fall in the numbers of heart attacks in British men in the last 25 years. The improvement is due to millions stopping smoking, better control of high blood pressure, and a big change in the pattern of cholesterol in the blood. However, the gradual rise in obesity in younger and middle-aged adults may change this for the worse as they reach their sixties. We look as if we are following the USA. There was a similar fall in heart attacks in North America until the late 1990s, but the obesity epidemic started sooner there, and there is now a U-shaped curve of deaths from heart attack. The Americans reached the bottom of the U around 2000, and numbers are rising again. We are about ten years behind them, so we can't be complacent.

Q: I had to be put on two different drugs for high blood pressure, plus a drug to lower my cholesterol. I'm only 51 and don't want to take them permanently. When will I be able to stop them?
A: I have no idea, and I expect your doctor hasn't either. The decision to stop either treatment will depend on how well they control your pressure and lipid levels, and whether they rise again after a trial period without them. That can't be predicted. However, taking medicines to lower your pressure and cholesterol is only a small inconvenience when you consider that they will substantially lower your chances of a stroke or heart attack. Since doctors in the UK started to manage blood pressure and blood fat levels in this way, strokes and heart attacks have fallen by more than half. Taking these drugs is a small price to pay for a longer and healthier life. Most people need to take them permanently.

Q: I'm 79, female, slim, and don't drink or smoke. I take bendroflumethiazide for high blood pressure. My last test showed it was a little up, and little different from previous levels. I don't want to take extra drugs, so what can I do to lower it myself?

A: As you don't smoke, have looked after your weight and keep fit for your age, you have already reduced the stroke and heart attack risks from your high blood pressure. So well done. At 79 you may not have to reduce your pressure by much, and your doctor may think that there is no need to meddle with it further by adding another drug. Your other risk is a high cholesterol level. You don't mention that, so ask about it, and see if you need to lower it along with your blood pressure, although the most recent research suggests that after 75 or so, a high cholesterol level may even be beneficial. So leave your doctors to decide on how or whether you should do that. In the meantime, enjoy a good quality of life, with healthy eating, and times set aside for exercise and relaxation each day. If your blood pressure remains high, your doctors may want to change your tablets or add one to the bendroflumethiazide. Much depends on their experience with your particular case.

Q: I have very high blood pressure that has not responded to drugs (I'm 29). I've been asked to go to hospital for a dye test in my veins. Is this safe, and how can it clear up my pressure problem? I have to starve from the night before – does this indicate I will have to be put under an anaesthetic?

A: The dye test is to see if your kidneys are working properly and that the blood supply to them is normal. Some cases of high blood pressure are caused by kidney problems, such as a poor blood flow to one of them. It is a very safe test that has been done for many years. You won't need an anaesthetic: the starving for 12 hours beforehand is to make the test less complicated and to empty the bowel, so that the picture is clearer.

Q: I had high blood pressure during my two pregnancies. That was 15 years ago, and my blood pressure hasn't been high since. Last week I had an insurance medical, and the doctor said that it was 'at the high end of normal' and my own doctor should be told. Why is this? I feel fine, and don't want to go on long-term tablets if I don't have to.

A: There is some evidence that women who had high blood pressure in pregnancy are at higher than normal risk of having strokes in later life. The chance of stroke is directly related to the height of the blood pressure. So you should have your blood pressure checked regularly, and if it remains higher than normal you need to take treatment to bring it down. That's why the insurance doctor gave you this advice. Do take it. If you need to take blood pressure lowering drugs, then follow your doctor's advice on that, too. You can't tell what your blood pressure is yourself without having it measured. It doesn't necessarily give you any symptoms – until you have your first stroke.

Q: I was told six months ago that I have high blood pressure, and have been taking bendroflumethiazide since then. Unfortunately the pressure level hasn't changed much and the doctor is thinking of adding another drug. I don't feel ill. Is it really necessary for me to go on more drugs?

A: It is very important to bring your pressure down into the normal range. If it remains high you are at greater than normal risk of a heart attack or stroke. That's what your doctor is trying to avoid for you. The fact that you don't feel ill doesn't matter. Your first symptom of illness could be your last – one-third of all people who have heart attacks or strokes don't recover from their first attack. Keeping blood pressures down with drugs has lowered the numbers of deaths from these two devastating illnesses by more than 40 per cent in the last 20 years. So you must take your doctor's advice.

4

The skin

Q: I'm confused about the sun. We are told not to sunbathe because it causes skin cancer, then to sunbathe because the extra vitamin D protects us against heart attacks and internal cancers. What should we do?

A: Sunbathing is fine as long as you don't *burn* (tanning is a form of burning in fair-skinned people). Your skin cancer risk rises with each episode of burning or tanning. On the other hand, we make vitamin D from the reaction of sunlight on the skin, and lower than average vitamin D blood levels put us at higher risk of heart attacks than if they were normal. (For purists the cut-off point is 15 nanograms per millilitre – the source is the long-running Framingham study in the USA.) Taking vitamin D improves your survival if you have cancer of the prostate, breast or colon, but paradoxically, there are more of these cancers per head of population in countries at low latitudes, in which you would have expected much more exposure to the sun. We Brits get most of our vitamin D from food – fish, other oily and fatty foods, including supplemented dairy products – so sunbathing isn't our only source of it. The message is to enjoy the sun sensibly, not just for the vitamin D but also for the sheer pleasure of its warmth. Don't we all need it in January?

Q: I've had a small lump on the inside of my upper left arm for a few months. The doctor said it was probably a cyst and booked me for a scan but it disappeared before the appointment day. It returned shortly after, and is pea-sized (it had been larger). It isn't painful but it can feel uncomfortable, and can itch. Should I get it checked out again?

A: Definitely, if only for your peace of mind. A small lump that comes and goes like this is usually an inflamed lymph gland or a subcutaneous cyst, and it is probably benign. But you need to have it examined and perhaps even removed for microscopy. The first step is to go to your doctor again – remember that he/she thinks it has gone and needs to know that it has returned. Your doctor will assess whether it is hard or soft, freely mobile in the tissues around it or fixed to them, whether or not it is tender, and also whether there are other similar lumps elsewhere that you haven't noticed (yes, it can happen!). So be prepared to have a thorough physical examination, which could involve your neck, armpits, groin, abdomen and breasts, as well as the lump. All this is meant to reassure you – and also your doctor, so don't be at all alarmed.

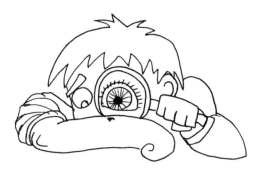

Q: I've had a cracked and chapped upper lip for over a year. It's flaky and itches, and is worse in winter. I've been told it's due to stress but my only stress comes from having this ugly lip. Can you help?

A: Please see your GP about this. A persistent lesion in your lip needs investigation to rule out a physical cause before it is considered stress-related. Presumably you aren't constantly biting the cracked area. Two possibilities have to be faced – a local lesion in the lip itself, which may be infected or due to a small benign growth, or something wrong with your general health. A year is too long to wait for an answer. The first step may be for you to ask your doctor about seeing a dermatologist. A general health check may be appropriate, too.

Q: I'm 28 and play a lot of sport – football in the winter and cricket in the summer. I had what I thought was a patch of eczema on the top of my foot. It was itchy and red, and just looked like the eczema I had as a boy, so I used some hydro-cortisone cream on it. That seems to have made it worse, and it has spread. Could it be athlete's foot, and did I make a mistake putting hydrocortisone on it?

A: Yes to both questions. Eczema as a child doesn't usually arise out of the blue again when you are adult. And athlete's foot is far commoner than eczema on the feet. Steroid creams make fungal infections like athlete's foot much worse. Ask your phar-macist for advice on athlete's foot, unless it's a raging infection, when you would be better showing it to your doctor.

Q: Eczema started on my ankle, and has spread up my leg. It has appeared on my arms now. A tube of steroid cream hasn't helped. What should be my next step?

A: Do you have varicose veins? If so, they may have caused it to start on the ankle. They will have to be treated before the eczema will clear away completely. I'm curious why it spread from the legs elsewhere. This suggests not eczema but contact dermatitis or a skin infection. You need to find out more about it, which means your doctor will probably refer you to a spe-cialist clinic.

Q: I'm thinking of having botox surgery to remove wrinkles. How long do the effects last?

A: Between three and six months. Then the muscles that have been paralysed by this enormously powerful poison recover, and the wrinkles return. Surgical removal of wrinkles, like a turkey neck, lasts a year or two longer. If you are a smoker they will come back a lot faster, as the chemicals in the smoke begin to destroy the skin again. If you have stopped smoking, then you have a better chance of looking like one of those ancient Hollywood actresses in your seventies. You have to consider then whether that is appealing or appalling.

Q: For eight years I have had dermatitis in my face and scalp. I have had dozens of creams containing different steroids that just make my skin even redder. It is getting worse. Can you suggest something?

A: It sounds as if you need investigations to find out the cause, which can range from fungal infections (which steroids will make worse) to allergies or a form of acne. Have you had scrapings taken from the affected area? Have you seen a dermatologist? It is unusual to prescribe steroids for any prolonged period for the face, as this can lead to reddening and thinning of the facial skin.

Q: We are hoping to go on a sunshine holiday with our children. However, our toddler son has eczema. Is that likely to get worse or improve with the sun? Can you advise us?

A: Eczema usually improves in sunshine, but keep him cool when it is hot, and get him to wear a wide-brimmed hat and loose cotton clothing as well as a sun block to prevent sunburn. A T-shirt that you can keep wet – he will find that fun – will cool the skin and prevent or relieve itching. Enjoy your holiday.

Q: I have had skin tags for many years now, but they are becoming quite grotesque. I have several on the eyelids, along the side of my face, chin and neck and would so like to get rid of them. Is there a solution?

A: Yes, and a fairly easy one. You can have them removed either surgically (usually under local anaesthetic) or (for the ones further from the eyelids) by liquid nitrogen. Your GP will gladly arrange it for you.

Q: My partner and I have cut out meat and dairy and we're convinced we have more wrinkles. Could there be a link between our diet and ageing?

A: I don't know of any. But if you are eating too little protein (and you have lost your two main sources of protein from your diet) you may be losing some elasticity in your skin. Elastin, the substance that keeps your skin supple, is a protein. Lose that and wrinkles surely follow. Check your diet with your GP, who will advise you on what you may be missing. You may even need to have your blood protein levels checked. You didn't mention whether or not you smoke. That is the commonest cause of accelerated wrinkling with age. Of course, the wrinkles may just be your natural ageing process, and the link with food just a coincidence.

Q: Why are some moles raised and some flat – is one type more risky than another?

A: 'Moles' are more properly called pigmented naevi, and most of us have quite a few of them (up to several hundred) if we look carefully enough. Some remain flat, like freckles, some are thicker than the surrounding skin and become raised above it. Most of us have the odd 'dermatofibroma' on our skin, perhaps on a leg or an arm. It is a small dome-shaped firm lump, that may or may not be pigmented (it's often pink), around two millimetres in diameter.

The vast majority of moles, whether flat or raised, are and remain harmless. Of course, the recent publicity about the sun and skin cancer has raised doubts about this statement, and people are constantly aware of the slightest change in their skins, especially if they have at some time had sunburn. So what are the changes that mean things have taken a turn for the worse?

Here are the latest guidelines from the American Cancer Society and Cancer Research UK on when to worry about a mole possibly becoming malignant, and progressing to a 'melanoma'.

There are three major signs – changes in size, shape, and colour – and three minor signs: inflammation, crusting or bleeding, a feeling that it is different, or is painful, or itches, and a diameter of 7 millimetres or more.

All these changes can start in a flat or a raised naevus, or in a dermatofibroma, so be alert to them. Usually a malignant melanoma has an irregular, rather than a smooth edge, and the depth of the black, brown or blue colour varies across the surface, but if you have a mole with one or more of the 'majors' and one of the 'minors' above, you must see your doctor about it.

Above all, get to know your skin, so that you can detect a change in any part of it. How well do you really 'know the back of your hand'? Shut your eyes and try to picture it – the length of your fingers, the shape of the veins and tendons, the spots and hairs in your skin. Then open your eyes and see if you were anywhere close. You will be shocked by how far out you were. So look at your skin once in a while and see if you could remember the pattern of moles. There are astronomers who can look at the night sky and can, at a glance, pick out a new star, say a supernova, that wasn't there the previous night. It shouldn't be so difficult to do the same for your skin.

Q: I am an 88-year-old woman and would like to know what I can do for dry skin on my legs and feet. Sometimes the fronts of my legs are shiny and red from the top of my foot halfway up the leg. The backs of my legs are flaky, and under my feet is rough. I also have a dry mouth although I drink quite a lot of water and only have an odd pot of tea. I occasionally drink a small carton of fruit juice and eat one piece of fruit a day. I take Fosamax once a week for osteoporosis and betahistine three times a day for vertigo. I have a small spoon of cod liver oil and malt a day.

A: The most likely diagnosis here is a skin infection, probably a fungal one, like athlete's foot. The flakiness and roughness under the feet give the main clue. However, it would be stupid of me to diagnose at a distance. You must see your doctor, who may take scrapings (they don't hurt) from the affected area and send them to the local lab for identification. Scrapings may not even be needed, as sometimes the nature of the infection is obvious. However, your skin problem may also be a side effect of Fosamax. Your doctor will want to check on this possibility, too. You may have to change the Fosamax for another treatment. Do not treat this yourself: you do need a check-up.

5

Nutrition and the gastrointestinal system

Q: I'm travelling to the Far East on business and don't want to offend my hosts by refusing their food. However, monosodium glutamate (MSG), which seems universal in Asian food, gives me migraines and vomiting, forcing me to bed for up to two days. How can I prevent this happening, other than starving myself?
A: You must avoid foods containing MSG. Prescription drugs do prevent migraines and the upset gut, but are not as effective as you would like. You can only explain very tactfully to your hosts how MSG affects you. In the Orient, hosts are usually very sensitive to their guests' dietary needs, and they will surely be pleased to offer you MSG-free meals that you can eat with confidence.

Q: I often have indigestion when I go out for dinner or drinks with friends, even if I consume less than I might at home. The main difference is that I talk more when I'm out. I become incredibly full, find it difficult to take even a sip of water and my nose starts to run. Lying down eases the pain but isn't usually possible until I get home. After a few hours I feel sufficiently sick to gag, which brings up only air, and then I feel better. I can't burp but it sounds like I need to. Everyone else seems able to eat, drink, talk, dance: why do I have so much trouble?
A: It sounds highly likely that you are an air swallower. When you socialize you constantly gulp down small amounts of air – it's a habit that you don't notice yourself, and as the air accumulates it becomes a large bubble in the top half of your stomach. Hence the feeling of fullness and the change when you lie down – the bubble isn't then pushing up against the under-

side of your diaphragm. It is easy to diagnose, but much more difficult to manage, because it's so hard to stop this involuntary swallowing. The more you think about it the harder it can be to stop. However, recognizing that you have the problem is the start of the eventual cure. When you are chatting, try to avoid swallowing, or at least to postpone it for some time before you do. We produce saliva constantly, and it has to be swallowed from time to time: you are simply doing it more often than most and taking in air as you do so. It's a matter of training yourself to do it less. It takes time, but you should be able to do it.

Q: I often wake up to a pain in the left side of my stomach and back, between my hipbone and the angle between my ribs and my spine. Going to the loo or passing wind relieves it, but it can recur throughout the day. I seem to be bloated, too, from time to time and a bit tender in the same area. Is this likely to be irritable bowel, and should I just treat myself? I feel absolutely healthy otherwise. I'm 55, female and this is new to me.
A: Please have a medical check. You may be correct that your symptoms are due to cramps and trapped wind associated with irritable bowel. It is the likeliest explanation, but there are other possibilities. They include backflow of urine from the bladder to the kidney, diverticular disease (in which pockets of gas form in small 'blebs' on the surface of your bowel), or other bowel disease that is causing partial obstructions. The symptoms may even have an ovarian cause. Your doctor will want to rule out all of these possibilities before concluding that you have irritable bowel. So you need to be examined, and perhaps have further tests, such as abdominal ultrasound and even endoscopy. You need to know the cause of your symptoms before treating them.

Q: I get a churning feeling in my stomach. I've been examined and my doctor says I'm not to worry, that it is just an irritable bowel and that I'm getting cramps. However, how can I stop worrying? I think I have cancer, and I'm not being given tests.

A: Believe your doctor. Irritable bowel is the commonest diges-tion-related complaint. A huge number of people sent to gastroenterology clinics have it, and for the most part, they have to live with it. If they were all investigated, they would take up far too much valuable time that should be spent on people who really are suspected of having cancer. If you truly are ruining your life worrying about it, then your doctor may arrange for an ultrasound examination and perhaps an endos-copy to deal with your concerns – but if that has a normal result, please take that as the final word.

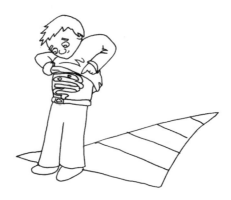

Q: I'm 56. I have a constantly bloated and painful tummy. I don't have much appetite, but I'm not losing weight. I've been told I have irritable bowel syndrome, but treatments haven't helped much. Now I read that the symptoms might be explained by early ovarian cancer. How can my GP check on that? I'm very worried, but I don't want to waste his time.

A: We GPs have been asked to look on bloating in over-fifties women as a possible 'red flag' sign of ovarian cancer, and to examine and investigate accordingly. It involves abdominal and pelvic examinations, vaginal ultrasound and a blood test – measuring the CA125 antigen. Please see your doctor who will, I'm sure, take things further. You may well just have IBS, but you will need solid reassurance about your ovaries. If you wish to know more please contact <www.targetovarian.org.uk>, the website for the charity Target Ovarian Cancer.

Q: Please settle an argument for us. Are fast foods in restaurants really more fattening than the food we cook at home?

A: The Americans think so – in fact in 2008 cities like New York and San Francisco enacted 'calorie-posting' laws for all restaurant menu dishes to try to educate diners on how fattening foods can be. California has since made the laws state-wide. The study findings that led to this action were astonishing. A fruit smoothie, for example, gives the consumer 1,180 kilocalories, and a single pizza portion over 2,000. The average restaurant customer consumes 1,000 kilocalories, yet adults need only around 2,000 for a whole day. The UK Food Standards Agency would like pubs and restaurants here to give more information about the fat, sugar and salt content of their food, but only on a voluntary basis. Legislation seems far off, but what the Americans do, we seem to follow a few years later. The answer for us, in the meantime, is to know what we are eating.

Q: What's the best way to treat a tongue that is burning from eating a chilli that's too hot? Drink water or beer?

A: Neither. Slosh a lot of milk around the inside of your mouth. The burning sensation is caused by molecules of capsaicin (found in all chillies and responsible for the hot feeling) binding to taste receptors on the cells on the surface of the tongue. The proteins in milk will strip the capsaicin off the receptors and ease the pain. Water or beer won't do this – all you will do is temporarily cool the tongue, but the heat will return very quickly, because the capsaicin is still there.

Q: Is it true that eating spicy foods (made with hot chillies) will increase your risk of cancer?

A: No, it isn't. In fact there's research evidence that it may help to cure it. Capsaicin, the active chemical in chilli peppers, actually kills cancer cells grown in laboratory culture. While it seems to have no effect on normal cells grown under the same conditions, it kills cancer cells by two different mechanisms – they either explode or shrink. For purists, the first effect is on the cancer cell mitochondria, and in the second it seems to command the cells to 'commit suicide' by a process called apoptosis. In a few years we may be using it as an anticancer medicine. In the meantime we already prescribe creams containing capsaicin (made from peppers) to alleviate the long-term pain after shingles. It works by 'deadening' the pain nerve endings in the area of skin affected by the illness.

Q: If chillies protect against cancer, is there less of it in countries where a lot of chillies are eaten, say in India or Central America?
A: Difficult to say, I'm afraid. The problem is that in these countries there are environmental causes of cancer, too, like repeated exposure to other chemicals or excess tobacco and alcohol use that will complicate the picture. I'm not sure that the research has been done to prove things either way.

Q: My mother used to swear by camomile tea as a painkiller and in reducing temperatures when we had sore throats or flu. Is there any proof that it works, because it does seem to soothe my children when they have coughs and colds?
A: I grew up in a camomile-loving family too, but always thought it was an old wives' tale. I may have been wrong. Camomile, green peppers and celery may be effective anti-inflammatories. They all contain luteolin, a substance that has been shown in the laboratory to reduce inflammatory reactions in the brain. It is now under research as a potential treatment for brain diseases in which inflammation may be involved. Alzheimer's and Parkinson's disease are two; viral meningitis and encephalitis may be others. In the meantime, keep drinking the camomile and, in addition, eating celery and peppers.

Q: We are always being advised that salt is bad for us, and to cut it down. But can eating too little salt be harmful? What are the symptoms of having too little salt?

A: In developed societies like ours, there's probably no chance that we will eat too little salt. There is salt in so many foods that you would have to be dangerously faddy to avoid it, and you would become deficient in proteins, minerals and vitamins as well. You wouldn't then know which symptom was due to lack of salt and which due to the other deficiencies. In the less developed world there are isolated mountain valleys where people eat far less salt than we could possibly do. They are just as healthy as people in nearby valleys where the rocks and soil contain more salt. People with rare kidney diseases, or for whom mistakes in drug treatments (sadly it happens) have made them salt deficient, feel sick and dizzy, have low blood pressure, and may lapse into stupor or even coma. However, that would never happen to a normal person who is simply cutting down on salt.

Q: I drink a lot of tea without milk, usually piping hot. Is it true that it could raise my risk of cancer of the oesophagus? A friend suggested that there was new evidence that it does.

A: That evidence is from a *British Medical Journal* report of a study in northern Iran, where some people drink tea at temperatures above 70 degrees Celsius. The results are solid because they aren't complicated by other possible cancer-inducing factors such as alcohol or smoking, and the researchers measured the temperatures of the tea as it was drunk. There were twice as many oesophageal cancers, proportionately, in people who drank their tea 'very hot' than in those who drank their tea lukewarm. There's a simple answer to your dilemma: let the tea cool for only five minutes after brewing it, and you will lower your risk to average levels. Don't stop drinking tea – it has health advantages that counterbalance this single piece of evidence from Iran.

Q: What is the difference between irritable bowel and inflammatory bowel disease, which my doctor refers to as IBS? Are the two the same?

A: No. Inflammatory bowel disease describes two main bowel disorders, ulcerative colitis and Crohn's disease. In both there are ulcers in the bowel wall, and there is diarrhoea with blood and mucus (like phlegm) in it. In irritable bowel the bowel wall is healthy: the problem is a form of cramps in the bowel muscle. That leads to pain and distension in the abdomen with wind and occasional bouts of 'rabbity' stools or constipation. There is no blood in the motion. The two forms of bowel disease are quite different, with very different treatments.

Q: We hear a lot about whether tea or coffee can be good or bad for you. What's the medical consensus?

A: The balance of studies suggest that they are beneficial rather than harmful. Tea and coffee in themselves are not nutritious, in that they don't give you calories you can use for energy. But they do contain plenty of chemicals which if you were given them in a pill you would classify as drugs. Tea, for example, contains flavonoids that in theory protect the heart and brain against 'free radicals' – damaging chemicals that arise as a result of disease or ageing. The initial Dutch studies of 'frequent', 'seldom' and 'never' tea drinkers found that men who had consumed the most flavonoids (in apples, tea and onions) had the least heart disease. Other studies agreed that people who drink at least three cups of tea a day have around 10 per cent fewer heart attacks than non-tea drinkers. Cancer prevention studies haven't been consistent, perhaps because drinking very hot fluids may actually lead to cancers of the oesophagus. We shouldn't drink our tea or coffee too hot.

Coffee doesn't protect you against heart attacks in the same way as tea, but nor does it promote heart disease, as people once thought it might. One odd result (from over 51,000 Norwegians) was that people who drink more than three cups of coffee a day are less likely to die from cirrhosis of the liver than those who drink none or just a little. However, if you have an alcohol problem don't make that an excuse to drink more coffee and keep on boozing.

Q: My friend takes vitamins A and E. She says they are antioxidants that prevent cancer and heart disease. Is she right, and if so what is the right dose? I'm thinking of taking them – I'm 50 and a healthy male.

A: Although they are antioxidants, several long-term and large trials have shown that extra vitamins A (such as beta-carotene) and E do not reduce heart attack risk. In fact, some of the trials were even stopped because there were more deaths in the vitamin groups than in those given a placebo. A *Lancet* editorial in 2002 reviewed all the evidence and strongly discouraged adding them as supplements, as we get enough of both vitamins from a normal diet. That appears to be the orthodox view still – there have been no convincing new studies to reverse it. I don't understand why people still promote such supplements.

Q: I use around ten tablets of a sweetener, Canderel, every day. It says on the label that it may contain phenylalanine. What is the risk of taking it? Is phenylalanine harmful?

A: Canderel contains two sweeteners – maltodextrin, which is related chemically to sugar and is harmless, and aspartame, which is a chemical that tastes extremely sweet, but is unrelated to sugar. The note that it is a 'source of phenylalanine' is simply a warning to the very small number of people who have a condition called phenylketonuria, and who must avoid phenylalanine. They know who they are (they have had the condition since birth) and you are obviously not one of them. For everyone else, phenylalanine is an amino acid, one of the 'building blocks' of protein that we all need. It is part of our normal food and is not dangerous in any way.

I'm more concerned about your use of sweeteners. If you are trying to slim, they can be counter-productive. You need to lose your taste for sweet things, and by swallowing ten sweeteners a day you are constantly reinforcing it. You will then find it difficult to resist other sweet foods – and they will keep your weight up. Change your drinking habits by drinking weak tea with a slice of lemon, and no milk, sugar or sweetener, and see how you get on. Try coffee without sweetening it, too. You will get the real taste of the tea and coffee, and begin to like it. In a few weeks you will wonder why you wanted to sweeten them.

Q: A friend is taking glucosamine for arthritis. Would it be worth me taking it? I have rheumatoid arthritis and diabetes, and my doctor isn't too keen on me taking it. What do you think?

A: In theory glucosamine is supposed to build up cartilage strength. That may be fine for osteoarthritis in which cartilage (the 'shock absorber' tissue inside joints) does deteriorate. I don't see how it can help in rheumatoid arthritis, in which the problem is an inflammation of the tissues immediately around the joints. So I tend to agree with your doctor, particularly as you have diabetes. When glucosamine is given to animals it raises their blood sugar levels, and although there are no studies to confirm this in humans, I would be wary of using it in someone with diabetes. The only study that has shown glucosamine to be of any value in humans is in knee joints – it hasn't been of proven help for pain or inflammation in other joints, and so far there has been no second study to confirm its effects on the knee. I'd want to see another one before I would recommend it. Glucosamine was removed from the list of drugs approved for prescription in most areas of the UK in 2009.

Q: How much does diet play in causing the pain of osteo-arthritis? Should I be avoiding any foods? I have arthritis in the hips and knees and don't want to have surgery.

A: There is no good evidence that avoiding any particular food will either prevent or treat osteoarthritis. Nor is it likely to do so, as it is a chronic inflammation of the joint surfaces, a tendency to which is inherited, and can be the result of repeated injuries or putting too much weight through the joints. Losing weight can help, as this takes the pressure off the affected joints. As for surgery, it changes people's lives, turning them from house-bound or chair-bound invalids into people who can walk and enjoy life again without pain. I'm amazed at the number of patients who do fantastically well after surgery. So don't reject surgery without a lot of thought about it.

Q: We have a lot of arthritis in our family. My sister says that eating a lot of fruit and vegetables can prevent it. Is this true, and what's the evidence?

A: The evidence came from a report in 2004 that looked at the eating habits of men and women in Norfolk. It reported that people eating very little fruit and vegetables every day were three times more likely to develop rheumatoid-type arthritis than those eating the most fruit and vegetables. It didn't make a difference to whether or not they developed osteoarthritis. So if your family arthritis is of the rheumatoid type, do eat a lot of vegetables and fruit. Of course, that's a good health tip for anyone.

Q: I have just been told that I have gout, due to uric acid crystals forming in my joints. How can I change what I eat, so that I can avoid this?

A: You can't avoid it completely, because uric acid forms nor-mally in your body after digestion of proteins found in a big range of foods. Some foods, like red meats and beer, are rich in these proteins, so you could help by cutting down on them, but there are effective drugs that help your kidneys to get rid of excess uric acid, and they can usually keep the symptoms under control.

6

Neurology

Q: My grandfather and an uncle died from Alzheimer's disease. What can I do to find out my chances? Would genetic testing help me?

A: Probably not. For example, having a negative test result for the genes that are linked statistically with a higher than normal risk of Alzheimer's wouldn't prevent you developing dementia in later years. And being given a positive result for them doesn't mean that you will develop Alzheimer's – it only slightly increases your chances. In an American trial reported in 2008, 162 non-anxious and non-depressed relatives of Alzheimer's patients were tested for apolipoprotein E (APOE) possession, a substance that has been linked to increased risk of the disease. Two-thirds were told their results and one-third were not (they were all volunteers, and accepted this beforehand). There was little difference in mood afterwards regardless of the result or of being kept in the dark, except that those given negative results were marginally happier than those given positive ones. As we don't yet know how to prevent Alzheimer's or how to reverse its effects once established, there doesn't seem any point in having the test.

Q: My 80-year-old father, who is physically fit, is forgetting things so that he has to write everything down. Is this dementia?

A: He needs a detailed assessment of his mental abilities before a diagnosis can be made. The doctor will want to rule out other illnesses, like low thyroid activity or depression, before dementia is diagnosed. The fact that he is writing things down himself suggests that he has some insight into his memory loss, and that he may just have age-associated memory deficit, which is normal, and not true dementia. Is there any intellectual loss, which is quite separate from memory loss? If so, then dementia is more likely.

Q: A relative has been dizzy for months. Her MRI scan did not find any damage to the brain. She didn't tell her specialist that she is also forgetful. She forgets, for example, making a cup of tea a few minutes before, then makes another one. Would Alzheimer's disease have shown up on the MRI scan? And would the specialist have tested her for Alzheimer's?

A: It's difficult to spot early Alzheimer's on any sort of brain scan. It is more easily diagnosed on memory testing. Her GP can do this, so it's important for her doctor to know about the memory lapses. She should talk to her doctor about her memory loss, or be taken by a relative who can describe what is going on. Alzheimer's is not the only possible cause of memory loss in the older person. She may be depressed, or even have an underactive thyroid – both of them eminently treatable, so it will be worthwhile seeing the doctor again if only to check on them.

Q: Can I be tested for my risk of Alzheimer's disease? I'm 53 and my mother developed it in her early sixties.

A: We don't yet have blood or other tests to predict risk of Alzheimer's. Researchers have studied the use of questionnaires designed to detect early stages of loss of memory and intellect in families with and without a strong history of Alzheimer's, but with no clear results. A small minority of predictions were accurate, but most of the subsequent cases of Alzheimer's weren't picked up. We may have to wait some years for more effective predictive systems. Maybe by then we will also have better treatments. If your mother was your only relative with Alzheimer's, your chances of early dementia are around the same as if you had no family history of it.

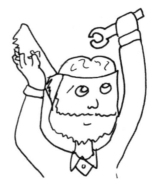

Q: My wife has multiple sclerosis and wonders about interferon treatment. What are the pros and cons? Does it really help?

A: In the early 2000s interferons were hailed as a great step forward for people with the type of multiple sclerosis that has periods of worsening (relapses) and improvement (remissions). Strong pressures for them to be prescribed for most MS sufferers were resisted by the NHS authorities because there was too little proof that they helped much, and the costs were high. The biggest review, of studies of 1,215 people with MS, found that although interferon did reduce slightly the numbers of relapses in the first year, there was no certainty that the benefit would continue after that. There were many drop-outs during the trials because of the drugs' serious side effects. The National Institute for Health and Clinical Excellence (NICE) therefore doesn't recommend interferon for MS. Yet for some people, it has pro-duced sustainable benefits. Everyone is an individual, and what works for some doesn't for others. As someone who practises in Scotland where there is a very high incidence of MS, I'm not bound by NICE, so we have some patients on it. But it isn't a miracle cure.

7

Smoking

Q: My husband smokes in the house – I don't smoke. He says that there's no real evidence that second-hand smoke causes harm, so I shouldn't be upset about it. What's your take on this?

A: Be upset. The latest evidence is so clear that even FOREST (the pro-tobacco lobby) can't argue against it. After Scotland banned smoking in public places in March 2006, admissions to hospital for acute coronary attacks fell by 17 per cent. (They had been falling by around 3 per cent before that.) In the same time, in England and Wales, without a ban, the fall was only 4 per cent, a hugely significant difference. Crucially, the fall in admissions was greatest in people who had never smoked and in women – in other words, second-hand smokers who were no longer exposed to smoke in public places. Their blood cotinine levels (the best measure of exposure to tobacco smoke) had fallen in line with the drop in heart attacks. No one could argue against a

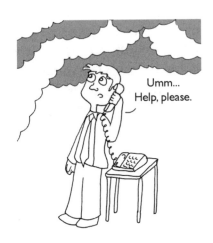

Umm...
Help, please.

link between the two. A 2010 report stated that passive smoking contributes to 1 per cent of all deaths.

Q: I've been smoking since my teens. I'm 58, and have been told I now have chronic bronchitis. Is there any point in me stopping smoking now? Surely the damage has been done.

A: Smoking puts carbon monoxide into your blood and heart muscle, nicotine into your arteries and brain, tars into your lungs, and cancer-inducing chemicals into your throat, lungs, kidneys and bladder. If you stop, in one day you will lose the carbon monoxide, lowering your risk of heart attack. In two days the nicotine will be gone, lowering your risk of stroke and gangrene in the limbs. In three months the lungs will be free of tar, lowering your risk of lung cancer and easing your bronchitis. And in six months your risk of new cancer starting in the throat, lungs, kidneys and bladder would be reduced by nine-tenths. And you ask if there is any point in stopping? If what you are doing to your body weren't so tragic, your question would be laughable.

Q: Is it true that smoking cannabis is less harmful than tobacco or drinking?

A: No. Most people smoke cannabis mixed with tobacco, so that you get the harmful tobacco anyway. Cannabis itself has been linked with a particular type of lung disease in young people – called bullous lung disease, in which the lungs become filled with balloon-like cysts, leading to early lung failure. Heart attacks have been reported as more than four times more likely to happen within an hour of smoking cannabis than at any other time. Smoking cannabis is a major risk to your health, even when you leave aside the effects it has on your brain. Finally, cannabis smokers take a much larger volume of smoke in with each puff, hold their breath four times as long and have five times the carbon monoxide in their red blood cells than cigarette smokers. No one should play down its dangers.

Q: Is it true that there is a link between smoking and developing diabetes? Smoking has been blamed for lots of diseases, but isn't diabetes going a bit too far?

A: No, it isn't. Smoking is the health-destroying habit above all others. The follow up of 17,000 babies born in the UK between 3 and 9 March 1958 proved as long ago as 2002 that if you smoke during pregnancy you increase your child's risk of developing diabetes. It also showed that if you smoke as a teenager your risk of becoming diabetic rises. The news gets worse: if you continue to smoke after you develop diabetes you steeply increase your risk of heart attack, stroke, kidney disease and losing a limb due to gangrene. Enough said.

Q: What is the best way to stop smoking? Nicotine patches, gum or Zyban tablets?

A: They all help, but only if you are really determined to stop. If you are using one of them just as a prop, but still don't really see the need to stop, you won't succeed. I've found that when people really understand the terrible damage they are doing to their lungs and other organs by exposing them to the dangerous rubbish, poison gases, cancer-inducing and lung-rotting chemicals that are in tobacco smoke, they stop without the need for any aids. Every medical practice is now linked with a 'stop smoking' clinic. Join yours. That's the best way to give up tobacco.

8

Infection and the immune system

Q: What happens to our immune system as we grow older? Do we get fewer infections because we have had so many of them in the past, and are therefore immune to them? Or does it get less efficient, so that we have more infections? Please settle an argument for us.

A: I wish I could! Both happen to us. We have fewer colds because we preserve our antibody-producing reaction to them. The more colds we have had in the past, the fewer we will have in the future. But that doesn't work for all the infections and illnesses we are prone to. As we grow older our thymus glands (in our chest) shrink, and they can't produce as many T-cells (which kill invading infecting organisms) as they used to. And as we get older our white blood cells – the front-line defence against infections – don't work as efficiently as when we were young. Exercise boosts our responses to vaccines, although how it does so isn't understood fully. If we walk to the surgery for our flu and pneumonia jabs we should be better protected against

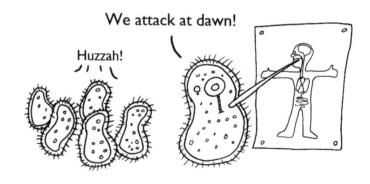

We attack at dawn!

Huzzah!

them than if we drive! So I haven't settled the argument. If you want to boost your immunity, then the easiest way to do it is to exercise regularly.

Q: I always get a cold and cough after a long flight. Am I imagining it, or is there a good reason for it?
A: We get several colds every year – probably several hundred in our lifetimes. That's because there are hundreds of different cold viruses to which we are susceptible. So when we have a cold after a flight it could well be coincidence – we were going to get it anyway. The theory was that the inside of an aeroplane with 300 people on board is perfect for spreading droplets of sneezes containing virus particles, and that if one person sneezes or coughs in the passenger cabin it is odds on that you will inhale the virus within a few minutes. However, tests of air quality inside cabins show that it doesn't carry any more germs than air elsewhere. We are just as likely to catch a cold wherever there are a few people around us as in a plane.

Q: Is there good evidence that current flu vaccines do any good?
A: Dozens of papers and surveys published regularly since the 1970s show that repeated annual vaccination of 'at risk' people with updated flu vaccines reduces their chance of catching it by about 70 per cent. It also reduces the severity of the illness in people who do catch flu in the winter after the vaccination. So it is as successful a vaccine as most. The problem comes when a new virus, with none of the surface antigens (used to make the vaccine) of the previous ones, appears. Before the swine flu outbreak in 2009–10, the previous time that happened was in 1968, when there were hundreds of thousands of cases, and thousands died. So it doesn't happen often, and today, when it does, the manufacturers seem to be better at fast production of the new vaccine. If you are on the 'at risk' list (your doctor will know if you are), it's definitely better to protect yourself against the

more modest toll of a non-pandemic year (in which there are usually several thousand cases) than not to do so.

Q: I've had a cough for a month, after a bout of flu. Do I really need to see a doctor, or will it gradually die down? When should we see a doctor for a cough?

A: If you are a non-smoker, any cough that goes on for more than two to three weeks needs investigation. Your doctor will want to look at your throat and nose, and listen to your chest and take things further from there. If you are a smoker, you will have a cough anyway. Stopping smoking should stop the cough within a month. If it doesn't then you need to see your doctor for an assessment of the damage you have done to your lungs. If you have a permanent cough and still smoke, talk to your life assurance company and your lawyer about your will, rather than your doctor.

Q: My neighbour gives her eight-year-old son echinacea every day to ward off colds and flu. She also gives him added vitamins. She says I'm neglectful of my children for not doing so. What do you think?

A: Colds and flu are virus infections that are passed from child to child (or adult) by inhaling droplets of saliva from a cough or sneeze. You are susceptible to the infection regardless of how much vitamin or any herbal or other medicine you have in your body. Echinacea does not kill viruses and there is no controlled trial to show that it protects against any infection. There are plenty of trials to show that in a developed country extra vitamins don't protect against these infections. So be confident that you are doing the right thing by your children. All you need to ensure is that they eat a good range of food, take normal exercise, get normal amounts of sleep, and are confident in their good relationship with you. Inculcating a habit of taking a medicine a day when you are not ill isn't good for your attitude to health when an adult.

Q: Why isn't everyone asked to wear face masks when there's a flu epidemic about – or even when they have a cold? Wouldn't they protect us when we are in a crowd? Why are doctors so much against them?

A: We are not completely against them, but they have very limited use. Doctors seeing lots of flu cases should probably wear them, but they become sodden after an hour and a half, so we would use at least six of them every day. As supplies of effective masks are low, we only use them when face to face with possibly infected patients. If everyone tried to use them, they would very quickly become unavailable for the key health workers who really need them. We will control the spread of infection far more efficiently by washing hands regularly, using tissues once only and disposing of them immediately and properly. Good hygiene is critical.

Q: We are going on a cruise, but have just heard that our ship has been affected by norovirus gastroenteritis. What is the likelihood of us catching it next month – about six weeks after it affected the passengers? We hear that that cruise was stopped, and the ship cleaned and fumigated.

A: Norovirus doesn't persist in the ship. It is transmitted from person to person in a fairly closed environment, like a hospital or a large ship. A passenger must have come on with it while infected, and the droplets of air from his/her breath, or the virus on his/her hands, did the rest. That's why cruise ships now insist on passengers using alcohol-based washes before they touch food, and each time they board the ship. It hasn't arisen from the ship's kitchen, which is almost certainly spotless. So enjoy your cruise – the chances of it happening again in the same ship are only the same as with any other ship, and if you take the right precautions you should be fine.

9

Exercise

Q: How much exercise should we really do every day to keep fit? And what is the advantage, if there really is one, of being physically fit, rather than just slim?

A: Physically we are still hunter-gatherers, despite a few thousand years of civilization. Hunters (the men) walked and ran around 25 miles a day, and gatherers (usually the women) walked around 20 miles a day. Once they had brought in the food they ate as much as they could as fast as they could, then slept for a couple of days until they were hungry again. So we're built to walk a marathon four or five times a week. No one can do that now, and the accepted wisdom is that an hour or so of brisk exertion (enough to make us breathless) three or four times a week is enough for us, as long as we don't hugely overeat like our ancestors in between times. As for the advantages of exercise, Swedish researchers have found that men who exercise regularly have a 30 per cent lower chance of developing cancer and are much more likely to survive cancer if they do develop it, than men of the same weight and height who don't exercise regularly. That's one big advantage.

Q: Does jogging harm your knees? I get pain at the side of the knee sometimes, and it worries me. Which other exercises are as good for fitness?

A: It shouldn't if you wear the correct shoes with cushioning under the soles and heels. It may do so if you already have an old cartilage injury or early arthritis. Pain at the side of the knee next to the other knee is common when you start and is usually just muscular strain. If the inside of the knee hurts, or it gets stiff, swells, gives way or locks, then you need to seek advice and to choose another exercise. Walking might be better (the shoes still matter) and swimming helps, though you have to swim for longer than you walk to get the same benefit. If you have bad knees, you will find breaststroke difficult; crawl and backstroke are probably better for you. If you prefer a bike make the saddle high enough to allow a near-straight leg at the lowest point of the pedal.

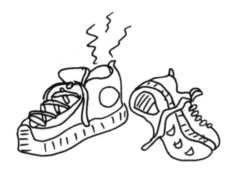

Q: I have been jogging regularly for the last few years, taking part in ten-kilometre and half-marathon runs. Recently I've had a pain in the middle of my left foot that is worse when running, but never really goes away completely even when I'm resting. Could this be a muscle or ligament strain, and what can I do to ease it? I don't want to stop my running unless I really have to.

A: You must see your doctor. It's possible that it is a strained ligament, but it could also be a stress fracture of a metatarsal, one of the bones in the centre of the foot. If that's the case (an X-ray may help) you will need to rest the foot. You may even have to have a walking cast for four to six weeks to let the fracture heal. After the cast is removed, you may still have to return to exercise slowly, say over four weeks, only starting to run again after that time, and then only if the foot is pain free.

Q: As I had an injury to my knee, I started walking/jogging in the swimming pool while wearing a buoyancy belt around my waist. I do this for at least 90 minutes a day on five or six days a week. I am 64 years old and I have found that this has not only improved my knee but my back pain is considerably less. Will this improve my cardiac fitness and how does it compare with the brisk walking I used to do on the treadmill for 30 minutes a day?

A: Yes, it will improve your all-round fitness, including your heart. It is precisely equivalent to a treadmill for 30 minutes a day, so keep it up. You might consider deflating the buoyancy belt, little by little, over the weeks until you don't need it.

10

The eyes

Q: I'm 22, have a healthy diet and exercise. But for the past year I've had dry eyes that are regularly bloodshot, and in one eye I have a permanent enlarged blood vessel. Prescribed eye drops haven't helped. Can you?

A: Could the clue be in your exercise? Are you regularly dehydrating yourself – not drinking enough fluids to compensate for the loss in sweat? Try extra fluids – drinking water when you're not thirsty, for example. If you have truly dry eyes you need to put the drops in every hour or so – perhaps you have used them too little. You may have a chronic conjunctival infection, so tests and perhaps an antibiotic ointment may help. If the dry eyes are linked to a dry mouth, then you may have Sjögren's syndrome, in which other secretions (in the gut, joints and vagina) are also less than they should be. That needs expert advice, so see your doctor again.

Q: I've just turned 50 years old, and have to drive a lot in my business. Recently I've found that I'm much more affected than I used to be by glare from streetlights and the sun. I can see all right to read and watch television without glasses. Is there anything I can do to help my vision while driving?

A: You need a full eye check-up. Increased sensitivity to glare could be the beginnings of a cataract – your lens may be clouding over. So see your optometrist for a full vision check, and visit your doctor for a full health check. Cataracts at your age may also be a sign of early diabetes or other conditions. You are due, anyway, at 50, for a well man check up.

I've got my eye on you, buddy!

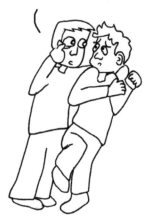

Q: What is 'lazy eye'? My three-year-old son has it, and has to wear an eye patch over it. How long will he have to wear it – and does the patch work? Will he have a squint?

A: His two eyes don't see equally, with the consequence that one starts to let the other dominate. The brain then relies on the vision it gets from the 'stronger' eye only. Eventually, if not treated, it will lead to difficulties in focusing, a squint, and perhaps double vision. So we put a patch over the good eye to force the weaker eye to focus and look for itself. Today we put the patch on for six hours a day over four months. That usually teaches the two eyes to work together, and will avoid double vision and squint later.

Q: Both my eyes water a lot. I'm told that my tear ducts are blocked, but my doctor doesn't suggest any treatment. What can be done for me?

A: It depends on how they are blocked. If it is due to catarrh from the nose, then that has to be treated, usually in the first instance with a decongestant spray. If the block is an actual narrowing of the ducts, then they can be opened by a surgical probe (although this is not always successful). If it is because your lower eyelids are lax (and are folding outwards) then they can be repaired, too. So you need to talk more about it with your doctor.

11

Hands and feet

Q: My fingernails have lost their normal pink colour and turned white. I've also noticed my feet and ankles have swollen and I don't have as much energy as I used to. I'm 22 years old and female. Am I deficient in some vitamin, and if so, what should I take?

A: These are *not* the signs of vitamin or mineral deficiency. The combination of white nails and swollen legs suggests that you may have a serious kidney problem. It's called nephrotic syndrome, and is easily diagnosed from finding a lot of albumin in your urine. You must see your doctor as a matter of urgency. Don't try to treat yourself.

Q: I often get an incredibly cold right hand, while my left hand remains at a 'normal' temperature. Apparently the same thing happens with my feet. I'm male, 23 and have OK blood pressure. Any ideas?

A: If the problem were in the hands only, it could be easily explained. You might have pressure on the sensory nerves leading into the right hand – either in the wrist (that's carpal tunnel syndrome) or in the elbow, shoulder or neck. One unusual cause is an extra rib in the neck, putting pressure on the nerve as it leaves the spine. Your doctor would check all these possibilities. The difficulty comes when you mention the feet as well. That isolates any nerve trouble to the spinal cord itself – a much less common condition, and you would need a neurologist to pinpoint the cause. It's just possible that you have a form of Raynaud's syndrome, in which the small blood vessels in the skin go into spasm, leading to changes in how warm or cold you feel. If that were the case you would see a difference in the colour of the skin when you were cold – the fingers would go white. As you didn't mention a colour change I presume it doesn't happen like that. So give your doctor all the details on the times and occasions when you feel the cold.

Q: I'm 67 years old, and my older brother died suddenly from an aortic aneurysm in his abdomen last year at 70. My doctor has asked me to have a scan to see if I have one too. Do I really need one? I'm a lot fitter than he was and don't smoke – he smoked 20 a day. What are my chances of having an aneurysm?

A: About one in five, regardless of your smoking habit. Your doctor is right to ask for a scan. If you are found to have an aneurysm it is far easier to treat it before it bursts or leaks than to wait for an emergency. Aneurysms are weak spots in the wall of the main artery in the abdomen. About one in 20 men over 65 have them, but most of them remain below the size that would cause concern (under 5.5 cm in diameter). If you have had a near relative with one, the risk rises to one in five. The fact that you don't smoke is excellent, as you are more likely to have healthier arteries than your brother had. Don't worry about the scan: ultrasound is used. It is safe, painless and efficient.

Q: Do you have a cure for chilblains? During March I had very painful hands for the first time since I worked on bomber engines outdoors in all weathers 60 years ago. I can't think of a change in lifestyle that could have caused them. I'm otherwise fit and active. Now that the weather is warmer, my fingers are fine, but I would like to know how to protect myself against them next winter.

A: This is a really difficult one. Sometimes the simplest problems are the hardest to relieve. In cold weather, be sure to wear warm gloves and footwear, and to have a woolly hat covering the scalp and ears, and protecting the face. If any part of the body gets too cold, reflexes leading from it to the feet and hands shut down the circulation there, and chilblains follow. Some people swear by extra vitamin D as a protection, but there is no real evidence that any medication helps much. If you are taking a beta-blocking drug, that can make chilblains worse, so your doctor will help with an alternative. If you do get too cold, warm your hands and feet up slowly in lukewarm water at first, rather than toasting them by a fire or on a hot water bottle. Sudden reheating at high temperatures can make things worse.

Q: I'm 65 and have cramps in my feet, legs, hips and hands. Am I deficient in something? I don't add salt to food. Are there any cures or preventatives for cramp? Magnesium phosphate has been recommended for attacks and quinine for prevention – do they work and how do you take them?

A: Quinine as 200 mg of the sulphate or 300 mg of the hydro-chloride each evening is the usual treatment. Even then it only reduces the frequency of cramps by about a quarter. There's no other clinically proven anti-cramp treatment for the normally mobile person. There are more complex muscle anti-spasmodics for the cramps that complicate serious diseases such as multiple sclerosis or spinal cord injury, but they are not for you. You need to look at your lifestyle. Are you physically active, do you exercise regularly, eat a varied diet and keep well hydrated? Stretching your muscles with exercises and keeping them warm in the evenings may be the simplest way to avoid cramps. Extra salt isn't likely to help, unless you are over-exercising and sweating a lot. Occasionally cramps like yours are caused by a parathyroid gland problem, which changes the way calcium is used by the muscles. If they continue your doctor may check parathyroid function with a blood test.

Q: For the last two months or so I've been waking with very stiff knuckles and finger joints in both hands. It takes about an hour for them to loosen up. I think my wrists are swollen, too. My mother's sister had rheumatoid arthritis. Could these symptoms be the first sign of it in me? I'm female and 45, and have always been well until now. I've found that aspirin has helped a lot. Should I just take them every day, or should I see my doctor?

A: Please see your doctor. You may well be developing rheumatoid disease, and only a blood test, and perhaps some X-rays, will confirm it (or not). Aspirin or a similar drug may indeed be the best treatment, but you (and your doctor) need to know what it is.

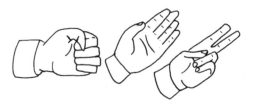

Q: I have lots of white spots on my nails. Is this a sign of lack of calcium? Are there other nail signs that we should be aware of?

A: The white spots are the outward appearance of tiny air pockets lying between the skin under the nail and the under-surface of the nail, usually caused by having knocked the nails against something. They don't have serious health consequences. Other nail problems, though, should cause you concern. Developing a spoon-shaped depression in the nail, so that you could hold a droplet of water on it, is a sign of iron deficiency: anaemia. That can have many causes, so if your nails are spoon-shaped, get a check-up. If you have small red flecks like tiny lines under the nails near the tips, see your doctor. These may be small 'emboli' (thromboses in small blood vessels) from a heart problem. Tiny ridges that run lengthwise from cuticle to tip don't, as a rule, matter much. They are just the way the nails grow in some people. But if the ridges are at right angles to the growing direction of the nail, this may indicate times of ill-health (the nails have stopped growing for a short time) and you should ask for a medical.

Q: I have a fungal infection in the nail of my big toe. My doctor has given me a paint to put on it for three months. Why does it take so long to cure it?

A: The nail grows very slowly, and it is difficult for the treatment to penetrate into the nail deep enough and in enough concentration to kill the fungus. At least the modern treatments do work – in the past once a nail was infected it remained so for the rest of your life.

12

The ears

Q: I've become hard of hearing recently (I'm in my seventies) and wonder if the digital hearing aids that you can buy from the companies advertising them in the press are worth the price. They seem to cost a lot of money – several thousand pounds. Are they effective, and do you think they are worth the money?

A: Not at that price! Several companies have made digital hearing aids available through the NHS at prices below £100. Get advice from your doctor about your hearing before considering 'going private'.

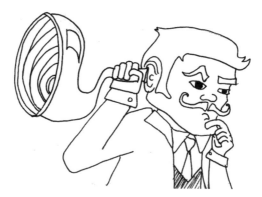

Q: About twice a week I have the sensation that I am in a chamber in which the sound is distorted. It lasts a few minutes, then goes away. My doctor says my blood pressure is OK. Could this be catarrh in the ear? And would cutting out dairy products help? I'm 58.

A: Without a comprehensive examination of your ears, nose and throat it's difficult to say what this might be. It could be coming from blockage by mucus in your Eustachian tube, which passes from the back of your throat to the inner side of your eardrum. The problem could be deeper in the ear, due to high pressure in your inner ear. However, that is likely to go along with tinnitus (a constant noise in the ear) and with loss of balance. You may need a specialist examination to sort them out. There's no evidence that dairy products are linked to either, especially as the symptoms have started in middle age.

Q: I've had tinnitus, on and off, lasting a day or two at a time in both ears, for around two years, after an attack of labyrinthitis. In between attacks I have no problem. How can I get rid of it? Would cutting out milk products help?

A: I don't know of any established link between tinnitus and types of food. You don't sound as if you have classical tinnitus (ringing or rushing noises in the ears), which is usually present all the time. You may have an intermittent blockage of your Eustachian tubes. They equalize the pressures between the back of your throat and the inside of your eardrums. If they are blocked, say with mucus secretions, that could be the source of the tinnitus. As this is curable, see your doctor, who may refer you to an ENT specialist.

Q: I have sticky brown wax that regularly needs syringing away, and my wife has dry, scaly pale wax that just falls out. She never has to have her ears syringed. Is it something I'm doing wrong?

A: No. You have simply inherited different genes for earwax. People with 'wet' earwax have a gene that makes the cells lining the ear 'push out' oils that condense into wax. People with 'dry' wax possess a mutation in the gene that stops the 'pumping action' of the cells, and stops the oil production. Japanese researchers looked at the genes of 244 people with different types of wax, and worked out that the mutation for dry earwax occurred millions of years ago in north-east Asia and spread southwards and westwards from there. So your earwax problem isn't because you wash your ears differently from your wife, nor did you do anything to cause it. You were born to have your ears regularly syringed, and your wife wasn't.

Q: Do big ears help people to hear better than smaller ears?
A: Our ears aren't independently direction-finding like those of bats or deer: we have to turn our heads to find the direction of sounds, so the size of the outer ear is less important than in other animals. A few people can wiggle them, but not to any useful extent. They play only a minor role in collecting sound waves, so that smaller ears collect sound and channel it towards the outer eardrum just as efficiently as larger ones. It's when the sound passes through the eardrum and is magnified by the three bones in the middle ear that the process of hearing efficiently really starts.

Q: Three weeks ago a heavy box fell on the crown of my head, which seemed to sever or 'shock' something in my right ear. Since that very instant, I can hear only muffled sounds on this side, and as a musician this is extremely alarming. There has been some improvement over the weeks since, but it is by no means good enough. I have had no headaches, or pain of any sort in areas such as the shoulders and neck. Is there anything I could do to improve the situation? Should I see a specialist?
A: Yes, definitely. You need to know how much damage you have done to your hearing and if it is 'nerve' damage or 'conduction' damage. You may even need to have a skull X-ray to check on any fracture around the middle and inner ears. Your doctor will send you to the appropriate ear clinic. There is nothing you can do yourself, but as a musician who depends on her hearing for her living you should get the utmost of attention and expert advice – and only a specialist can do this.

13

Hernia

Q: My husband is about to have an operation for a hernia in the groin. How long will he be in hospital, and when is he likely to be back to work? He is self-employed and can't afford to be off long.

A: Most hospitals now do most of their hernia surgery under a local anaesthetic as a day patient, so he should be home the same day. Some prefer to keep people in overnight, but that is getting rarer as the results of day hospital surgery are proving to be excellent. It's usual for an office worker to be back at his desk after two weeks, but if your husband does manual or heavy work he should take a full month off, just to make sure that the repair of the muscles has completely healed.

Q: Does lifting heavy weights cause hernias? I developed one after helping workmates to shift paving slabs. Would that be more than a coincidence?

A: You must already have been predisposed to develop the hernia because of a defect in the muscles of your abdominal wall. The heavy lift may, by raising the pressure inside your abdomen, have pushed a loop of gut through the defect. In men the commonest site for the defect is in the groin, where the tube from the testes enters through the abdominal wall. So you had a hernia waiting to happen – you simply induced it by the strain of lifting the weight. I'm afraid that if you are looking for compensation for an injury at work, you wouldn't get much sympathy in a court!

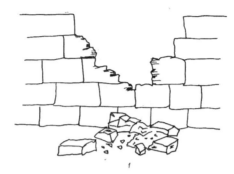

Q: I've had a large hernia in my right groin for years. I am really not keen on surgery, and have used a truss to keep it under control. Is there any harm in doing this or must I face the knife at some time? It used to disappear completely when I laid down at night, but it is still obvious now when I lie flat. Does that make a difference to whether or not I should have surgery?

A: Everyone with a hernia should consider surgery. Any hernia can suddenly 'strangulate' – which means that the loop of bowel inside it can twist on itself, depriving itself of blood supply and therefore oxygen, and blocking further progress of its content through it. So you can suddenly develop both obstruction of the bowel and gangrene of the bowel wall. This is a serious, life-threatening emergency that has to be operated upon imme-diately, when you are far from your best, physically – often in shock. The fact that it no longer disappears when you lie down suggests that there is so much bowel in it now that it can't return through the gap into your abdomen. That indicates you are at serious risk of strangulation. See your doctor immediately.

Q: My wife has been diagnosed with a hernia near her navel. We thought that only men had hernias. What has happened in her case?

A: Both men and women can have small defects in their abdominal muscles that can lead to hernias. Obviously inguinal

hernias (in the groin) are commoner in men because of the connection with the tube from the testes, but men and women have
equal chances of having hernias elsewhere. Your wife was almost
certainly born with this slight problem, and it has come to her
notice only recently perhaps because she has been straining
her muscles. One woman patient of mine, a housekeeper in a
large hotel, developed hers after lifting a big bundle of laundry.
Another felt hers for the first time when pushing her husband's
car in a snowdrift! Your wife may be able to relate her first aware-
ness of something wrong to a similar incident. Happily, hernias
in sites other than the groin are less likely to have serious complications – but they still need to be operated upon.

14

Women's health

Q: I'm 19, and am thinking of going on the pill for the first time. I've always been healthy, don't smoke, and am not overweight. My mum had a problem with a blood clot when she was taking the pill and doesn't want me to start. What are my chances of developing a thrombosis, and is there a particular type of pill that would minimize them?

A: The most recent results are from the Netherlands and Denmark, and they are equally relevant to British women. The Dutch found a slight increased risk of leg vein thrombosis (with a lesser, but still raised, risk of lung involvement) on the combined oestrogen/progestogen pill. The risk was greatest in the first three months, and decreased as time passed. The type of oestrogen in the pills mattered: those containing levonorgestrel were least likely to be linked with thrombosis. Progestogen-only pills and intrauterine hormone-releasing devices did not raise the thrombosis risk. The Danish study found that the extra risk was tiny: a thousand women would have to take the pill for a year to give one extra case of thrombosis. As a non-smoking young woman living healthily, your risk is extremely small.

However, it would be best to find out exactly why your mother had her thrombosis. Was she older than you are now when she had her episode? Was she taking one of the older high-oestrogen pills? Was she a smoker? Did she have high blood pressure or an abnormal cholesterol profile? Was her clotting system normal? Your doctor ought to know, so that you can make the correct choice for yourself, taking the family history and your own life-style (which may be different from your mother's) into account.

Q: I get a pain in my right groin and hip. It starts just before my period, and comes on for a few days before it goes away. I'm in my late thirties. Must I see my doctor?

A: Yes. It could be caused by cramp or inflammation in the womb, by endometriosis (a problem with the womb lining) or by a small fibroid. It could even come from the right ovary. You almost certainly need an internal examination and perhaps an ultrasound test to find the cause. Ask for a longer than usual surgery appointment, and let your doctor know all about the pattern of your pain. Preferably organize the appointment at the time you have the pain, but before the period has started.

Q: I've just been told that I have breast cancer. How can I get in touch with other women who have had it, and find out how they coped? I've heard a lot from my doctor and nurses, but they haven't been in my position.

A: A number of websites may be of help to you. One is the Association of Cancer On Line Resources (ACOR) at <www.acor.org>, which has contributions from survivors, carers and doctors and covers over a hundred diseases. Another is the charity DIPEx, whose website is at <www.healthtalkonline.org>. This organization is the brainchild of Dr Ann McPherson CBE and Dr Andrew Herxheimer, who have both been ill themselves, and lets people share their experiences of health and illness. Both sites are extremely helpful to people who are, naturally, struggling with coming to terms with their illnesses. Do talk to your doctor or specialist nurse, too, about how you are feeling. They may be able to put you in direct touch with your local Cancer BACUP service, which provides excellent and sympathetic support.

Q: My wife, who is in her fifties, has recently had a mastectomy for breast cancer. One of her friends in a similar situation in a different part of the UK simply had the cancer removed, and was allowed to keep her breast. Was this because different surgeons have different approaches, or because my wife's cancer was different from her friend's? She is disturbed by the thought that she might have kept her breast.

A: Breast cancer surgeons throughout the UK follow strict guidelines about whether they can treat a cancer by 'lumpectomy', as your wife's friend has had, or by mastectomy, which involves removing the whole breast. The decision depends on how big and how active the tumour is, where it is in the breast, and to what stage it has spread. When your wife was offered a mastectomy it would have been considered the most effective treatment in trying to ensure that all the cancer was removed and to reduce the risk of a recurrence to an absolute minimum. Each woman is different, and needs a different pattern of treatments. Be reassured that good quality of survival is just as likely with either treatment. Your wife may be offered breast reconstruction surgery later.

Q: My wife has postnatal depression after our first baby. She has never been depressed before. We have lots of support and she is recovering slowly, but both of us are worrying about what may be ahead. How long is she likely to be depressed, and is she more susceptible than normal to bouts of depression in the future?

A: Most women with postnatal depression who, like your wife, respond to treatment, recover completely. Some are particularly susceptible to depression after childbirth: they have around a 40 per cent risk of another depressive episode after subsequent pregnancies, but it seems specific to a pregnancy. They have a lower than usual risk of becoming depressed outside the context of pregnancy and birth. On average postnatal depression lasts for between three and six months, although some women still have a low mood for a year or more. So you can both be optimistic: knowing these figures can help you plan, but be sure to follow your depression team's guidance in the meantime. It is obviously working well.

Q: My daughter started lactating when she was 16: it lasted for months then petered out. At 26 she has started lactating again. A blood test showed that the hormone responsible was at a normal level. Why is it happening and is there any need for concern?

A: The medical term for lactation that hasn't been preceded by pregnancy is galactorrhoea. It's fairly common in teenage as the breast matures, and usually settles as your daughter's did. Its recurrence ten years later may be just as benign. It can be a complication of some contraceptive pills, especially if she has taken them for years. The hormone tested was prolactin, which is produced by the pituitary gland (inside the skull) to induce milk production. Its normal level strongly suggests that her pituitary is not the problem, and that the breast tissue may just be extra sensitive to it. Higher prolactin levels point to a benign tumour in the pituitary gland. She should talk to her doctor about the results, and if the milk is bothering her, ask for a specialist opinion. She may be offered bromocriptine, a drug that blocks prolactin levels and stops lactation. It does have side effects, and she needs to weigh its pros and cons with her doctor.

Q: I'm a woman going through the menopause. I don't want to take HRT because of the risks. What do you think of black cohosh? A friend suggested I try it.

A: In 2004 the Committee on Safety of Medicines in the UK advised general practitioners against the use of black cohosh. This was on the basis that ten UK women had reacted badly to it, seven of whom developed liver disease. Two needed transplants because the damage was irreversible. Why not talk to your doctor about how best to control your menopausal symptoms? There are plenty of relatively safe and effective treatments.

Q: I take both thyroxine for an underactive thyroid gland and HRT for menopausal problems. Sadly, I have no sexual feelings. Is one of these treatments to blame?

A: It is unlikely to be the thyroxine: that should make you more active, physically and mentally. Your HRT may not be suitable: it can sometimes lower your sex drive. More likely than that, however, is that something apart from your medication is worrying you, and this is affecting your sex life. Can you talk it over with your partner or your doctor?

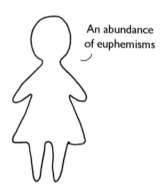

An abundance of euphemisms

Q: I have one breast bigger than the other. Why is this?
A: We aren't designed to be exactly symmetrical. Look at the two halves of your face. Split your face down the middle, make a mirror image of each half, stick the mirror images together and you will see two people, who vaguely look like you, and who look even less like each other. It's similar for breasts – we can't expect the breast on one side of the chest to grow to be exactly the same as the other one. They can differ in volume by around a third. Which one is the bigger is decided simply by chance, and not, for example, by whether you are right-handed or left-handed.

Q: At 37 I've started to get a hairy chin. I'm female, so that disturbs me. What is happening?
A: Part of this may be due to a subtle change in circulating hormone levels, as the normal ratio of oestrogen to progesterone (the two main female sex hormones) changes with age. With rising progesterone and falling oestrogen, you are more

likely to grow excess hair. At the same time your production of testosterone, the male hormone, remains level (women do secrete testosterone) so that its influence on your hair growth (and your libido) is heightened. It's sad that a sex urge surge, so to speak, coincides with the appearance of a hairy chin.

Q: Why do we women live longer than men?
A: Could it be because we men look after your every whim, and die early from the stress that imposes on us? I wouldn't dream of suggesting such a sexist and condescending answer. Sadly, men are born with a big disadvantage. The Y chromosome that differentiates them from women carries little else but sex chromatin (the protein that determines that men have the dangly bits). It's a tiny apology for a decent chromosome. On the other hand women have two X chromosomes, fully resplendent with a host of goodies other than their sex proteins. That gives females the edge in all sorts of ways – extra strands to their immune systems and being immune from a host of illnesses. That X chromosome advantage alone explains why women live, on average, five years longer than men, if they manage to survive into old age. Lifestyle also matters. Women who never marry tend to live longer than married women. Bachelors die younger, on the whole, than married men. I wonder why?

Q: My wife has been diagnosed with an inactive thyroid. What does this mean and what are the consequences?
A: Your thyroid gland is wrapped around the front of your larynx, your voice box. It produces thyroid hormone under the control of the pituitary gland, which hangs by a stalk from the base of your brain in a neat cavity in your skull. The pituitary gland secretes thyroid-stimulating hormone (TSH) into the bloodstream, where its rising levels are picked up by the thyroid gland. It, now stimulated, then sends out thyroid hormone into the blood. The more active your thyroid in its response to TSH,

the faster your pulse, the faster you think, the more physically active you are, and the hungrier you are.

An overactive thyroid leaves you thin, hungry, physically active and mentally alert, with a fast heartbeat and wide open eyes. An inactive thyroid is the opposite. If you fail to produce thyroid hormone, then you slow down, mentally and physically. Your heart rate falls, you think more slowly, so much so that it has been confused with dementia, your features coarsen, your hair falls out, your skin thickens, and you put on weight even though you don't have a particularly good appetite. If your thyroid gland does pack up we replace the missing thyroid hormone by a simple pill. The dose is determined by how you respond and you need to have blood levels taken of the hormones and of TSH every few months to make sure that you are still OK.

An inactive thyroid is usually due to an 'autoimmune disorder' in which the body's immune system thinks that the gland contains 'foreign material' that must be destroyed. The mistake is a costly one, leading to eventual destruction of the cells that produce thyroxine. It isn't lethal, and modern treatment is extremely effective.

Q: I have osteoporosis. I was told to take a pint of milk a day to increase my calcium levels, but a friend says that will put me at risk of a heart attack. What's the answer?

A: Some friend! Is he or she qualified in giving such advice? A pint of milk contains enough calcium to maintain your bone calcium level each day – so it will help your osteoporosis. And a pint of skimmed milk actually contains more calcium than a pint of whole milk – so you can drink that without consuming too much fat and without increasing your heart risk. Eat plenty of leafy green vegetables as well – they will also boost your calcium levels. And exercise as much as you can: that will help keep up your bone strength too.

Q: My wife and I want to start a family. She is very slim, weighing only seven and a half stones and being five foot five tall. She doesn't want to put on weight, because she says she will 'balloon' if she does. Will being underweight lower her chances of conceiving?

A: She is at least a stone underweight, and this may well lessen her chance of becoming pregnant. However, much depends on why she is too light. Does she exercise a lot, yet eat normally, or is she starving herself, in a minor form of anorexia? If it is the first case she has a better chance – but she should still try to put on weight before she conceives. Women who are poorly nourished during pregnancy tend to give birth prematurely to babies who are underweight for their delivery dates. So please discuss this with your wife and see if she can change her attitude to her weight.

Q: Is it true that if women want to conceive they shouldn't be too thin? My son's partner is very thin, yet she does want to start a family. Would she be better to put on a little first?

A: Women who want to conceive should eat healthily. If they are underweight when they conceive they tend to give birth prematurely to underweight babies. However, you, as her partner's mother, may find it difficult to persuade the lady of that. Tread warily when you discuss such things. A very tactful chat with your son might help, perhaps to persuade them to get advice from their doctor. She may not be as underweight as you think: perceptions of weight have changed recently, as the population has become much more obese generally. So be very careful in how you talk to her.

Q: How can I know that my menopause is starting?

A: For most women the menopause covers a few years from start to finish, the time varying from woman to woman. The medical definition of the menopause is the time when the periods stop, but that's not easy to determine. Some periods stop suddenly, others become further and further apart until they eventually stop without the women knowing exactly when the last true period was. That's difficult for contraception: I've known two women in their late forties who assumed, because they had had no periods for over six and nine months respectively, that they were now past pregnancy. They weren't: fortunately both welcomed their new babies, as did their twenty-something brothers and sisters!

A rule of thumb for when to expect the menopause is that if you started your periods early, say at around 11 years old, you can expect them to go on longer, say until your late forties. If they started late, they may end a few years earlier. But this is such a rough guide that it can't really be a forecast for each woman individually. Your mother's age at menopause might be a better guide, but only if you enjoy the same lifestyle as she did. For example, smoking makes a difference – smoking women on average start the change several years earlier than non-smokers.

Q: I am distressingly flat-chested, and am considering having implants – not large ones – simply to give me a figure that makes me feel more like a woman. However, my father's sister and a maternal aunt had breast cancer. Do implants increase my chances of later cancer development?

A: Be reassured. The latest and longest study, of 6,200 Scandinavian women with breast implants, that started in 1963, showed no link between the surgery and subsequent raised risk of breast cancer. Naturally your surgeon will examine your breasts first and make any necessary follow-up appointments, but any future change would, in theory, happen regardless of your surgery. Do talk to your doctor about your family history: you may be referred to your local specialist for a risk evaluation and advice.

15

Men's health

Q: Two months ago I discovered I had a small lump in my penis, about halfway along it. Now my erection is painful and is bent, so that intercourse is very difficult. It is definitely not a sexually transmissible disease. What is this, and can it be treated? Could it be a tumour?

A: You almost certainly have Peyronie's disease, in which the shaft of the erect penis develops a permanent bend around an area of scar tissue. It can be treated by specialists, so see your doctor about it. Don't be embarrassed: your doctor will understand. It is neither sexually transmitted nor a tumour, so you can be relieved on both counts.

Q: I've decided to have a vasectomy, but I hear that some men have pain for a considerable time afterwards. Is this true, and what are the chances of it happening to me?

A: Most men go through an uncomfortable few days after the operation, but it settles, so that after a week they are without pain. However, around one in 20 may develop what is known as post-vasectomy pain syndrome, or PVPS. We don't know what causes it: a nerve may be trapped at the site where the tubes are tied. Men who have PVPS may need nerve blocks or even, in a small minority, a reversal of the vasectomy to relieve the pain. The fact that a few men develop it shouldn't put you off.

Q: For nearly two years sitting down has been painful, just behind my testicles and in front of my anus. Prostate and testicle scans are normal. I go to the gym several times a week, and am otherwise very fit. Could my exercising be a cause?

A: It's possible. You may have strained the muscles between

your coccyx (the bottom end of the spine) and your perineum, the area you describe. It could have happened after a fall. These tail-end muscles take a long time to heal, so you may just have to wait until it gets better.

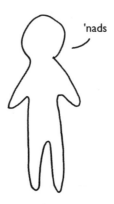

'nads

Q: Is it true that eating something in tomatoes prevents prostate cancer? My husband doesn't like tomatoes, but would be willing to take a supplement of the substance concerned instead. His father had prostate cancer.

A: Lycopene, a chemical found in tomatoes, has been shown to lower the risk of prostate cancer. But whole tomatoes or tomato concentrates are much more effective in doing so than just taking an extract of lycopene. He would be better to start liking tomatoes. If he can't bear them as a fruit, use whole tomato pastes, sauces and juices in your cooking, as in pastas, soups and pizzas. By the way, just because his father had prostate cancer doesn't make him particularly prone to it – very few cases are inherited. However, he should talk over his fears with his doctor, who may want to reassure him with a blood test for the disease.

Q: I've been told that I have benign prostate enlargement. Will I have to have an operation, or can it really be treated with prostate-shrinking drugs as my doctor says? I haven't been sent to a surgeon, which worries me.

A: About one in five men between the ages of 50 and 65

have symptoms relating to this form of prostate enlargement. Imagine the waiting list times if they all had to be operated upon. The whole NHS budget would be used up just in prostate surgery. Happily, we have effective drugs designed to shrink enlarged prostate glands. We only consider surgery if the prostate is infected, bleeding or causing long-term retention of urine in the bladder, with back pressure on the kidneys. So be happy with your initial treatment. You will be followed up regularly to make sure you don't need surgery – do attend your follow-up appointments.

Q: I have had a lot of trouble passing urine since a prostate operation four months ago. Do I have to just bear it, or should I ask for a further opinion?

A: Prostate operations are supposed to clear up this trouble, so there must be some complication. This can be anything from an infection in the bladder to an irritable bladder, or the fact that the prostate has grown again. So you need another assessment from your specialist.

16

Genetic issues

Q: My fiancé and I have only recently discovered that we are related through our great-grandfathers, who were brothers. We know, of course, that cousin marriages put children at risk of inherited illnesses. What are the risks for third cousins like ourselves? We still want to marry, but should we risk having children?

A: First-cousin marriages do put children at risk because they increase the chances of children carrying two recessive genes that can lead to illness. This risk is much diminished, but not quite down to the risk between non-related partners, with each generation away from the common ancestor. So a three-generation difference will carry a tiny extra risk. If you are worried, you can always ask for advice from your local genetic institute: your family doctor will give you the address. However, in Iceland, where the isolation of the population has led inevitably to relatives marrying, there may have been advantages for distant cousin partners. There, in studies of cousin and non-related marriages between partners born from 1800 to 1965, the marriages of third and fourth cousins were the most successful in rearing healthy children. It appears that 'genetic compatibility' conferred by carrying similar genes outweighed the small risk of developmental disasters.

Q: We are blue-eyed parents who have a brown-eyed child. A friend says that's impossible, which naturally upset my wife. What has happened?

A: In school biology lessons we learned that eye colour was very simply inherited. We were taught that there were two genes for eye colour, one for brown and one for blue. The brown was dominant, the blue was recessive – which meant that if both or just one of your genes were for brown, you had brown eyes, and only if you had two blue genes would you have blue eyes. So if both parents have blue eyes, neither possesses the brown gene and their child would have blue eyes. This was wrong. We now recognize seven shades of eye colour from very light blue to very dark brown, with shades of darker blue, green and hazel in between. The colour differences depend on several genes, not just two, and the mix can mean that a baby can have almost any eye colour regardless of the colour of either parent's eyes.

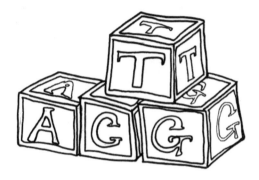

Q: Why do I get flushed and headachy after only a little alcohol, while others can manage to drink a lot more than me without ill effect? It isn't fair.

A: Alcohol is broken down in the body by an enzyme called alcohol dehydrogenase. Many alcoholics possess a particular variant of the 'alcohol dehydrogenase' gene that makes them tolerate much more alcohol than other people, allowing them to drink more than is healthy without feeling the ill effects that others do. However, anyone with any mix of genes can become alcoholic, suggesting that it is social circumstances, rather than basic body biochemistry, that matters most of the time.

There is one exception. A few people have a form of another gene, 'aldehyde dehydrogenase', that makes them sick and ill after drinking only a small amount. They soon learn to avoid more than the minimum of alcohol, and don't become alcoholic. Sounds like you are one of them. Maybe you are one of the lucky ones. It may not be fair, but you have the bonus that you won't become alcoholic.

17

Children

Q: I have friends who say that we shouldn't immunize our children with vaccines like MMR because our natural immune systems are more effective. What do you think? I got mumps and measles as a child and am perfectly healthy.

A: More accurately, you survived mumps and measles as a child. Every doctor of my generation watched children die from mumps and measles, and many more were permanently disabled by them. We also saw people die or be paralysed by polio, given permanently crippled chests by whooping cough, and die young from the effects of diphtheria-induced heart disease. In the 1920s tens of thousands of children died each year in the UK from infectious diseases. Thousands of babies were born blind, deaf and mentally disabled because their mothers had caught german measles (rubella) during their pregnancies. So there is absolutely no argument for the 'old-fashioned natural immune system'.

I can't believe that so many people have forgotten all this crucial history. Because these illnesses don't seem to be around, they think they don't need the discomfort of a needle to be protected against them. They listen to the people (we have had them since the eighteenth century) who oppose vaccination on biased spurious arguments that don't hold up. They don't heed the rational voices of the people who have studied the figures, done the crucial research, and are still watching people in the third world die from preventable diseases. In 2005 religious leaders in sub-Saharan Africa ordered their flock to stop vaccinating their children against polio, which was on the verge of eradication. The result was an epidemic of paralytic polio that, carried by one or two pilgrims, spread from Africa to the Far East, affecting tens of thousands of children and adults. It's still there, in a part of the world from which vaccination had banished it years before.

Here the allegations (made on very shaky claims by Andrew Wakefield, a doctor not a specialist in immunity) that MMR vaccination caused autism and bowel disease led to thousands of mothers in the UK and Ireland refusing the vaccine. Despite many studies refuting both claims and exposing the original research as wholly flawed, parents still refused their child the MMR vaccine. It resulted in a measles outbreak in the Republic of Ireland that killed two children, and another in the UK in the spring of 2006, killing one child and maiming many more. I would love the parents of the affected children to sue the doctor who started the anti-MMR campaign. I don't know why we still have the vicious anti-vaccination lobby here. Our colleagues in Europe watch what happens here and sadly shake their heads. The medical establishment has made its judgement on Andrew Wakefield: he is no longer able to practise in the UK.

Q: Our children get very car sick. What's the best way to help them?
A: Get them to pretend to drive the car. Drivers don't get car sick because they have to concentrate on the road ahead. If children can be persuaded to do that, then they won't get car sick, either. We use our eyes and our balance organs to know where we are relative to the space around us. Their pathways to the brain work together so that it gets the same message from both of them. When we are travelling in a car our eyes may be concentrating on something inside the vehicle, while the balance organ (fluid-filled semi-circular canals in the inner ear that act just like spirit levels) detects that we are moving on the road (or sea, or air, as the case may be). The brain gets confused – are we jiggling about in a car, or are we flowing along a road? – and

that causes the nausea and dizziness. To prevent that, persuade your children to coordinate their eyes and 'spirit levels' with the outside world, and not with anything inside the vehicle. In a car, that means looking at the road ahead. As it's often difficult to see ahead from the back seat, ensure that your children have good safety seats that allow them to see out. Playing games like identifying cars or lorries on the way helps them to keep looking outwards, and ban books and video games.

Q: Our 11-year-old son mirror writes, as well as writing perfectly normally at school. Does the mirror writing suggest he has a brain problem, or are there advantages in it?

A: He is in good company. Leonardo da Vinci and Lewis Carroll mirror wrote, and they didn't do so badly. It's thought that the ability is inherited, mainly by left-handed people. Instead of having one 'language' centre in one half of the brain, mirror writers appear to have two, one in each side, that are connected through the middle 'bridge', the corpus callosum, between the two halves. That means that they may have an advantage over the rest of us if they have a stroke, because they may retain the ability to speak regardless of which half of the brain has been damaged. They may also be better than the rest of us at learning new languages. So don't worry. There are advantages, and as far as is understood today, no disadvantages, for your son.

Q: Our 14-year-old son attends training for his football team, part of which includes a long run. Recently he has had to stop running for a while because of a pain in his right shoulder. Could this be his heart? He doesn't get it playing football, and he is otherwise well.

A: A right shoulder pain is unlikely to be to do with his heart unless he is a 'mirror-image' twin with his heart on the right side, rather than on the left. That's a chance in many thousands. It may be a 'stitch' caused by cramp of the diaphragmatic muscle, pain from which appears in the shoulder. Or he could be running with his neck muscles tense. If it's that, stretching and loosening his neck muscles before and during the run will help. He should see his doctor to make sure.

Q: Our five-year-old son has had a cough for a month or so. The doctor says it is asthma, although he doesn't wheeze, and doesn't struggle for his breath. Is this right? We think he may have a chest infection, rather than asthma, and should have antibiotics instead of an inhaler.

A: Many cases of asthma in children show up as a cough without obvious breathing difficulties. Your doctor will presumably have listened to the chest, and performed a 'lung function' test to confirm the diagnosis, so do accept it. A chronic chest infection causing a cough is quite different from asthma, and in any case an antibiotic may well not be needed. There is no stigma about asthma – around one child in six in some areas has it at some time. But admit your doubts to your doctor, to clear the air.

Q: Our infant son has Down's syndrome. We read that in the United States many children with Down's are given antioxidant and vitamin supplements to try to improve their intellect and prevent deterioration. Do they work, and why aren't they recommended here?

A: There is laboratory evidence that the nerve cells in Down's syndrome are more susceptible than usual to 'oxidative' damage, so antioxidants and vitamins, which in theory might protect against such damage, have been promoted. Sadly, a trial in which more than 150 British families participated has shown that there was 'no evidence to support' their use. The antioxidants used included selenium, zinc, vitamins A, C and E, and folinic acid: they gave results no different from a placebo. This latest evidence (2008) is the most convincing in a series in which vitamin and mineral supplements have failed to show any benefit.

It looks just like a human!

Oh sure, now he does.

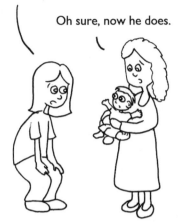

Q: My three-year-old grandson has serious difficulty opening his bowel. He screams in pain, doesn't pass a motion for two or more days, and when he does it is large and hard. He eats healthily and drinks plenty of fluid. What can we do?

A: He may have a small tear in the anus (a 'fissure') that hurts a lot when the motion is coming through it. Your doctor will need to examine him to confirm it or rule it out. He may be prescribed a softening agent, like lactulose, to ease the pain, plus a soothing ointment to be used before he tries to pass stools.

Q: In the past my children were given antibiotics for earache. My daughter's doctor won't prescribe them for my grand-children. Is that not putting them at risk of ear damage?

A: Today the official advice is that we should give only pain-killers to children with sore ears, the vast majority of which are due to viruses and get better on their own. Overprescribing of antibiotics in the past led to rising levels of bacterial resistance to drugs in the community, so that antibiotics did not work efficiently when they were really needed. However, if earache persists for more than 48 hours we then prescribe them. The result is that we only use around a tenth of the antibiotics we used to, without putting children's long-term ear health at risk.

Q: We are a bit confused about what we can give our children when they get fevers. Should we give paracetamol or ibuprofen? Both are heavily promoted for children with high temperatures. When should we use the one and not the other?

A: On the whole, we would only use one of them if children were distressed and uncomfortable – if they just have a 'temperature' but are not obviously ill or unhappy, then all that is needed is tender loving care. The drugs are useful in easing the headaches and muscle pains that come with a fever. As for which is more effective, so many studies show that they hardly differ that I don't prefer one to the other. We don't use ibuprofen in children with kidney problems or who are dehydrated, as it can put them into kidney failure. Nor do we use it in children who are susceptible to stomach inflammation, so we recommend paracetamol instead. For years we have avoided ibuprofen in children with asthma, but a comparison of it with paracetamol in 1,879 asthmatic children found no difference between the treatments in the number of asthma attacks afterwards.

Q: My grandson had meningitis when he was 11 months old. At five now, he is doing well in his first year at school. But what is the long-term outlook for him?

A: Some young children who have recovered from meningitis need to have special long-term care and attention to their behaviour in their teenage years. A study in 2003 of more than 700 13-year-olds who had had meningitis in their first year of life found that they were around three times more likely than others to behave badly at school and in the home. But this still means that most were perfectly normal in their behaviour and development. As your five-year-old is doing well now, there's no reason to think that there may be trouble ahead. The Meningitis Research Foundation would give you more information: your doctor will have the relevant number for your area.

Q: My daughter is always giving our granddaughter paracetamol for aches and pains. How dangerous is this? I'm worried that she might be harming her liver.

A: Parents today give paracetamol-containing medicines to their children much more often than your generation did. As long as your daughter sticks to the dose on the label it should be safe. Still, many families probably rush for the bottle too easily. If children have raised temperatures, cooling them down with a fan can be just as effective in easing their discomfort. If you do discuss this with your daughter be very tactful: don't take on the role of the interfering grandma.

Q: Some time ago the press reported on the possibility of dentists being asked to collect baby teeth from seven-year-olds, because they might be a source of stem cells. Did that ever come to fruition? As a parent I've never been asked by my dentist for my children's teeth.

A: I'm curious about that, too. Baby tooth pulp is full of stem cells, and there was a news item about harvesting them years ago in the medical press. It is a great idea, because it would be a good source of stem cells that would never run out and does not need any invasive or other unacceptable procedure to obtain them. I've tried to find out whether this has been taken further, but have had no success. There must have been some drawback that has stopped the research.

Q: Our seven-year-old thinks he is too big for his car booster seat, and wants to sit in the front beside his dad, on the normal seat. His dad doesn't see any harm in it, as long as he is strapped in. I'm frightened that he is still too small, and should stay in the back. Can you settle the argument for us?

A: The statistics strongly support you, not your husband. The commonest cause of death among four- to eight-year-olds is being inadequately restrained inside a car during an accident. Car booster seats are advised for children up to nine years old, and for smaller children beyond that age. Sitting in the front is a big risk if there is an air bag in front of the passenger seat, as this can suffocate a small child when it inflates. So keep him in the back on a booster seat for two more years at least.

Q: My 12-year-old son has had a lot of headaches, pains in his upper face and nose bleeds since he started his new school. My husband says that it is just nerves and he should keep on at school. I tend to keep him off when he is feeling bad. Which one of us is right?

A: He should go to school if he can, but I don't see how nose bleeds can be just nerves. He may have sinusitis, an infection in the cavities in the facial bones, so you should take him to the doctor to make sure. Do talk to his teacher, and find out if he is settling in at school. Your son won't tell you if he isn't! You could raise the possibility of bullying, which is common in first years in many secondary schools, if you think he is pleading a headache just to get off school.

Q: My 12-year-old daughter has developed arthritis in her knees and ankles, and has been put on methotrexate. It seems to be helping her a lot, but she has blood tests every week while on it. Must she really have so many tests? She hates the needles, and it's always a struggle to get her to go to the doctor.

A: I'm afraid she must. One of the side effects of methotrexate is a lowering of the white blood cell count, and that can cause her to be very susceptible to infections. The weekly test will catch any drop in the white cell count early enough to reverse it in time to keep her healthy. Her doctor may give you some anaesthetic cream to rub on the needle site before the sample is taken, to make it easier for her.

Q: We have just been told that our niece, aged seven, has developed acute lymphoid leukaemia. Obviously we are extremely distressed. Can you give a straightforward estimate of her chances of survival? A cousin died of it as a child in the 1960s.

A: It is impossible to comment on an individual case, but you can draw a lot of hope from the statistics. UK figures for survival from childhood leukaemias are among the highest in the world – more than 90 per cent. This is a fantastic achievement when we consider that 30 years ago they were nearly nil. So you have my sympathy, but please be optimistic.

Q: What are the risks of living near airports? We are moving close to Manchester airport and have three children aged from six to 12. Will the noise have a bad effect on them?

A: I wish I could say no to this question, but it's difficult to give a knowledgeable answer. Studies of people living near Amsterdam, Munich and Heathrow airports all suggested that there are problems for primary children living under the flight paths, mainly due to the repeated noise, and their schooling can be affected. One report is especially disturbing. After Munich airport closed some years ago, memory and reading improved in the schoolchildren living nearby. Then schoolchildren living near the new airport developed memory and reading difficulties within two years of its opening. It is also suggested that air near airports is polluted by particles of burnt aviation fuel ejected from planes taking off and landing. If you must live near to an airport, you would be better to commute to it from some miles away.

Q: When our son was five years old he developed Kawasaki disease, which was very frightening for us all. However, he recovered completely after a transfusion of immune globulin, and now, aged eight, he is very healthy. We were upset, however, to hear recently that transfusion of blood products like immune globulin might give people hepatitis C. Is this true, and what is the risk of our son getting it from his treatment?

A: It must be so close to zero that you can forget it. For the last 20 years, batches of human immune globulin have been produced with safety uppermost in the manufacturers' and doctors' minds. There has been no reported case of hepatitis C after its use in the UK. Thirty years ago, some mothers-to-be in Ireland were infected by a single contaminated batch given for rhesus problems. That was before the stringent rules for killing all possible viruses were applied to the way it was made. This must be the incident you heard about. Please don't worry. Be reassured that a recent survey of survivors of Kawasaki disease has shown that the vast majority lead completely normal lives.

Q: Is it true that taking probiotics every day will help children avoid eczema and asthma? A friend says that they could.

A: A single trial of one type of lactobacillus taken by women during pregnancy and then when breastfeeding, but only in families with histories of allergies, suggested that it partially protected against eczema in the babies. But it is only one study, and needs to be repeated. There is no good evidence that if probiotics are given to toddlers they will treat or prevent asthma or eczema. Sorry.

Q: Are dogs and cats in a house a danger or a benefit to babies and toddlers, say, for causing or preventing allergies? We have heard different opinions.

A: On balance, they seem to be more of a benefit than a hazard, despite the tragic occasional cases of dogs savaging small children. Some years ago a study reported that children in contact with two or more dogs or cats in their first year of life were less likely than others to develop asthma in later childhood. On the plus side, too, learning to deal with animals can help children develop their social skills. Naturally they should be taught good hygiene, and shown how not to provoke dogs into biting and cats into scratching. Female dogs and cats have the reputation of being safer than males in their contacts with small children.

Q: What is your view on the dangers of living near high-power radio, telephone or television transmitter masts? One has been erected less than a quarter of a mile from us, and we have three young children. We don't want to move, but should we do so for their sake?

A: Presumably you are worried about the possibility that exposing them to electromagnetic fields might stimulate leukaemia – something that has occupied a lot of researchers for years. The latest report is reassuring. German researchers found in 2010 that children living nearer than two kilometres to high-powered masts were not more prone to developing leukaemia than those living more than ten kilometres away from them. It is a well-conducted study using the case-control system, so its results are solid. Moving on account of a mast seems unnecessary, on this basis.

18

Travel

Q: How soon after an operation can you travel by air?

A: Much depends on the type of operation. For example, for some eye operations it can be six months. But it is a general rule not to travel by air within ten days after a major operation. If you have been bleeding from the stomach or gut that period extends to three weeks. After a stroke you can't fly for at least six weeks, and after a heart attack the flight ban extends to at least eight weeks.

Q: What's the best way to get over jet lag?

A: Going west is easier than going east. Westbound, keep awake as long as possible when you arrive, and go to bed at the normal time for your destination. After eight or more hours of sleep, you should wake fresh at the normal breakfast-time, and adjust quickly to the new time. Going east is more difficult as you have the disadvantage of losing a night's sleep before you start to adjust. You recover from the time change at a rate of only

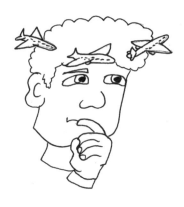

an hour a day. So if you have come from west coast America, an eight-hour difference, it takes eight days to be completely normal. Using sleeping tablets or stimulants to try to adjust faster can make things worse. Melatonin has its followers, but the evidence isn't impressive, and I'm not sure of its safety. I cope by accepting that I won't be right for a few days and taking that into account when making decisions.

Q: I'm thinking of going to West Africa for a beach holiday. Is it really necessary to have a yellow fever vaccination? I hear that it is particularly sore and there is a very low risk of catching it.
A: There was an outbreak of yellow fever in Senegal (near the Gambia) in 2008, with deaths numbering in the twenties. As there is no satisfactory treatment for yellow fever once you have caught it, I wouldn't go near West Africa without being immunized against it. The vaccine is no worse than any other immunization.

Q: We are off to Australia for the holiday of a lifetime in the New Year. What are our risks of getting a thrombosis on the flight? What precautions should we take?
A: It's difficult to express the risk without knowing your particular circumstances – some people are more prone to a clot than others. However, I presume you are healthy. In that case your risk of developing a venous thrombosis after a long-haul flight is 12 per cent more than if you were living at home. However, that risk is still very small, and amounts to 27 episodes of thrombosis for each million people taking a long-haul flight. Most of these go on to complete recovery. An Australian study reported that there is only one death from thrombosis after flights of more than 10,000 kilometres for every two million people travelling, and that might have happened anyway, regardless of the journey. You can help yourself lower even that risk by using elastic support stockings during the flight, getting up and walking around the aircraft regularly, doing muscle-flexing

exercises, drinking water regularly and avoiding alcohol. If you have a circulation problem, discuss your personal risk with your doctor in plenty of time before the flight.

Q: My son works in a game park in Africa and he has asked me and my husband to come out to visit him. He suggests that we take anti-malarial tablets with us. We are worried that they will have serious side effects. Do we really need to take them?

A: You either go and take the anti-malarial protection offered or you don't go. You would be crazy to go without it – the risk from malaria is far higher than the risk from the drugs. In 2003 a report in the *British Medical Journal* showed that although anti-malarials did produce side effects in 623 people travelling from Europe to Kenya and South Africa, none of these effects was serious. In the UK we see serious illness and deaths from malaria every year among people who did not heed expert advice. Your doctor will advise you on the right combination of anti-malarials for the region in which you will be travelling. I have been told anecdotally that there's less need to take anti-malarials in South African game parks than elsewhere, but as the UK authorities still recommend them I wouldn't go against that advice.

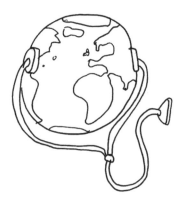

Q: We are going snowboarding later this month. Some friends say that we should wear protective helmets, others say that they can increase the risk of neck injuries. Who is right?

A: Definitely wear protective headgear. Snowboarding is a dangerous sport, involving falls on to icy and rocky surfaces, putting people at just as much risk of a head injury as cyclists and motorcyclists. Canadian researchers have shown that wearing a protective helmet reduces the risk of all head injuries by 29 per cent and of head injuries serious enough for the person to be kept in hospital by 56 per cent. Some people claim that wearing a crash helmet increases the numbers of neck injuries, but the figures don't bear that out. There were slightly more neck injuries in helmet wearers, but not nearly enough to offset the great benefit of protection against serious head injury.

19

Miscellaneous

Q: I have to avoid hot showers because they give me piercing headaches. What is the cause of this?

A: It is probably migraine. We have known for years that some people with epilepsy have to avoid hot water because it can bring on a convulsion. It's known as 'hot water epilepsy'. More recently the headache experts have advised us that there is also 'hot water migraine', which comes on only when you cover your head in a sharp flow of hot water. Your best way to avoid the migraine is to keep your shower temperature lukewarm. The fact that hot water seems to stimulate both epilepsy and migraine (but not, apparently, in the same person) has prompted research into a possible common cause, and perhaps may lead to new ways of treating both.

Q: My sister in America can buy melatonin without prescription to help her sleep. I'm told that here I would need a prescription, and that there are restrictions on its use. Why is this? My sister says it works for her.

A: Until recently melatonin hasn't been licensed in the UK, but one form of it has now been given the go-ahead. It can be prescribed only for three weeks, in patients aged 55 and older with 'primary insomnia'. That's because we see it as a drug, and the Americans, apparently, look on it as a supplement. The European Medicines Agency concluded from the trials so far that it has a small effect in a relatively small fraction of patients. It is probably about as effective as modern sleeping tablets (except that comparative trials haven't been done) with no obvious advantages except that it may cause less dependence and fewer withdrawal effects than others. There are several caveats – it shouldn't be given to someone with liver disease, or during pregnancy or while breastfeeding, and it interacts with several prescription drugs. If you smoke, it will have far less effect, and you can't combine it with alcohol. It is no miracle drug.

Q: A friend swears by a magnet that he wears to prevent rheumatism and depression. Could this really work?

A: Ever since electricity was invented doctors have tried to apply it to illness. The Victorians invented all sorts of sadistic shock machines to cure every illness, from malaria and tuberculosis to arthritis, melancholia (depression) and indigestion. The more lively the shock it gave the greater the claim for cure. Magnetism was seen as much more mysterious. You couldn't feel it, but you could see its effect on iron filings spread conveniently on a sheet of paper. That meant it had very particular powers. So every few years or so, magnetism gathers a reputation for healing, that has been refuted time and again. It seems that we forget the errors of previous generations. Google has more than 20,000 pages on magnetism and healing, but experiments comparing magnetic therapy with 'sham' magnets, in which the wearers did not know which were magnets and which were not, showed no difference in the results. The telling point for doctors like myself came with the use of magnetic resonance imaging (MRI) scans. Their very high magnetic fields have no healing or adverse effects: if magnets really did help our health, we would have expected people undergoing MRI scans to feel miraculously better!

Q: I take aspirin every day after a heart attack some years ago. I also get joint pains, for which I've been buying ibuprofen from the pharmacy. The pharmacist has now asked me to see my doctor, because he says the two drugs aren't compatible. Why is this?

A: Your pharmacist is following the advice from Dundee Medical School researchers who concluded that if you take a small dose of aspirin every day for angina or other forms of heart problem, you shouldn't take ibuprofen. Ibuprofen may act against the protective effect of aspirin on clotting and blood vessel walls – so you may be putting yourself at a higher than normal risk of a heart attack or stroke. Other anti-inflammatory drugs in the same group as ibuprofen don't have this anti-aspirin effect, so if you are taking daily low-dose aspirin, discuss with your doctor the drugs you can take, say, for those odd aches and pains or colds that everyone has from time to time.

Q: Is it true that if we are given antibiotics several times we get used to them, and they won't work if we get a future infection? **A:** No. It's not a case of our bodies 'getting used to them', but whether the antibiotic prescribed is the correct one to kill off your particular infection. It is not a question of whether or not you have had that antibiotic before, but only of whether the germ that is infecting you at this moment is susceptible to it. We can't 'get used to' an antibiotic – though bacteria can become immune to it. That's a different matter.

Q: For three years I've often woken up with a severe stiff neck, where I can't move my head to one side at all. It lasts for three to four days, is relieved only slightly by painkillers and there are no other symptoms. It has usually happened in the winter but I've had it this year in May. A friend's father mentioned that there could be a viral cause. Should I be worried? Could it be linked to shingles, which I had seven years ago? Another friend has mentioned a virus linked to chickenpox that causes mouth ulcers and general tiredness instead. Are they all connected? **A:** I'd better put you straight first about the viruses. Chickenpox (medical name varicella) is caused by a herpes virus that can reappear as shingles (herpes zoster) many years later. You can only have shingles if you have already had chickenpox. Cold sores are caused by another form of herpes virus – herpes simplex. It is unrelated to chickenpox and shingles. Shingles can leave people with lasting pain, but only in the area of skin affected by the rash – which I assume was not your neck. There's no evidence that a virus infection could lead to three years of symptoms like yours, so you have to look for another cause for your stiff neck.

The fact that you wake up with it suggests that your posture when asleep isn't right – is your pillow firm enough to support your neck while you are sleeping? One way to check is to balance it on your arm: if it flops down, it needs replacing with a firmer one that stays almost horizontal and that fits snugly between the point of your shoulder and the side of your head. Active exercises to stretch your neck may help to stop the stiffness: a helpful one is the first stage of the Alexander technique, in which you lie on the floor with your head resting on something firm, high enough just to tilt your chin down slightly, and then move the rest of your body away from your head. That helps to relax the neck muscles and prevent stiffness. Lie like that for about 15 minutes, if you can, three times a day. You may be surprised by the results.

Q: Since I started weekly swimming classes I leave the baths with a runny nose that leads to a heavy head cold affecting my sinuses and I have sore eyes, too. How can I avoid this? I don't want to stop swimming as I have had to stop running because of a knee problem. The pool uses an ozone system, rather than chlorine.

A: It sounds as if something in the water is irritating the delicate membranes lining your nose and sinuses. It may be related to the ozone system, but there may be other chemicals in the changing rooms or poolside (like cleaning fluids) that may irritate them. You could try using the nose pegs so popular with synchronized swimmers, and breathe through your mouth. And wear swimming goggles to protect your eyes, which have a direct connection with your nose through the tear duct system.

An antihistamine taken around half an hour before swimming might help. See your doctor about this – arrange the appointment when your nose is at its worst, so that it's easier to make the diagnosis and decide on prevention.

Q: Can you explain why people sneeze when they don't have colds or allergies? My husband sneezes every morning, several times, out of the blue, and I sneeze whenever I walk into bright light or look into the sun. What's going on?

A: For something so common, we know very little about why we sneeze like this. The nerve centre that, on stimulation, causes us to sneeze, lies in the area of the brain at the top of the spinal cord, the medulla oblongata. (People in whom it is damaged can't sneeze.) The centre is part of the 'parasympathetic' nervous system that helps to control the production of mucus in the nose and throat, the reaction of the stomach and gut to food, pupil dilation, heart rate, and blood flow to the sexual organs. In theory, when the parasympathetic nerves are in full flow this can produce a sneeze. So the bright light, drinking a whisky (one man's wife always knew he had sneaked a 'dram' when she heard him sneeze) or even orgasm can provoke a sneeze. There are lots of other nerve pathways packed into the medulla oblongata, so it's feasible that stimulation of them could also produce a sneeze. Presumably sneezes developed to clear nasal passages of mucus, but, like many biological mechanisms, they became the response to other physiological stimuli too.

Q: I've been taking a combined painkiller and muscle relaxant every day for years for back pain. They seem to help. Now my doctor wants me to stop them. Do I really need to?

A: Your doctor is worried about the long-term downsides of taking such drugs. One you may already have, in that you have become dependent on them. There is even a condition called analgesic-induced pain, in which people have pain actually caused by long-term use of painkillers. It's possible that your doctor suspects that you have it. Instead of taking painkillers every day, you may be better helped by a change in lifestyle. A lot of chronic back pain is caused by muscle cramps and spasms due to poor posture. Have you seriously tried relaxation and stretching exercises, or physiotherapy? Or an exercise such as swimming? Take your doctor's advice as an opportunity to assess your life and to approach your aches and pains in a different way.

Q: Our son is an athlete with hopes for the 2012 Olympic team. His coach has asked him to take vitamin and other supplements to build up his muscles. How do we know what is safe for him, and what may be construed as drugs?

A: Current Olympic athletes admit to taking vitamins, minerals, amino acids and other legitimate supplements. Whether or not they are beneficial over and above normal food intake is a matter of great doubt. I wouldn't recommend any of them, and would advise him to make sure he has a truly expert nutritionist on his team, and that his coach knows every rule in detail. Some legal supplements may help – for example, simple sodium bicarbonate has a reputation for preventing muscle cramps by neutralizing lactic acid build-up. I'm not even sure about that. And for me antioxidants, so popular with health magazines and complementary medicine promoters, are a no-no. There are two large-scale trials that conclude that they lead eventually to earlier death, rather than longer life.

Q: Can you catch cancer from someone else?

A: We can't catch cancer by having close contact with (living with or caring for) someone with cancer. However, non-smokers living with a smoker have a higher cancer risk than anyone living in a non-smoking home. Women with cervical cancer (cancer of the 'neck' or lowest part of the womb) may have caught it because they were infected with a virus (the human papilloma virus) years before. Starting your sex life early and having several partners makes you more likely to catch the virus, and to develop the cancer later. So women do catch cervical cancer, indirectly, from men carrying the virus without knowing it. The men have usually had no symptoms, though a few have had warts on their penises. Papilloma is the medical word for wart.

Q: I get a pain in my groin when I stand up, but it goes when I lie down. I'm male aged 25. My groin really aches after playing football, and sometimes feels swollen.

A: You may have a hernia. See your doctor: if it is a hernia and causes pain, the only answer may be surgery. The other possibility is a groin muscle strain – and that needs rest from football for a while.

Q: I have a pain in my left shoulder that comes on out of the blue at any time. It is as if something is 'jagging' me. Could you advise me on it?

A: I would need to know a lot more about it. Does the pain limit your shoulder movements? Is there a particular movement that brings it on? Does your shoulder ever 'stick'? Did you ever injure your shoulder? Are any other joints affected? Is your general health good? Are you losing weight? Do you have a cough? There are so many possible answers that you need to discuss all these questions with your GP. They are all relevant because shoulder pain can arise from a problem elsewhere such as the diaphragm, the lungs, the spleen, the liver, the heart and the spine in the neck. So do see your doctor and have a full examination.

Q: I have a very dry mouth, day and night. What can I do to improve it?

A: It sounds simple, but do you drink enough water? Sometimes just drinking a pint or two more water in the day is the simplest solution. However, there are other possible causes. One is dry mouth due to a shut-down in the production of saliva. This usually comes along with dry eye in a condition called Sjögren's syndrome. Another possibility is that you are on a medicine that makes the mouth dry, such as a blood pressure lowering drug or an 'atropine-like' drug for asthma. So if you are taking medicines, talk over the possible side effects with your GP.

Q: I'm 24. In the last few months my lower jaw seems to have grown, so that my face has changed. Would it be wasting my doctor's time to see her? I feel healthy, and have no other symptoms.
A: You must see her. Any facial changes after you have stopped growing can be a sign of general health problems or a particular problem in the bones of your face. Lower jaw overgrowth can be a sign of excessive pituitary gland activity, and that may have to be ruled out. If you have one, show your doctor a photograph of yourself before the change, so that a good comparison can be made.

Q: When I was a child I developed a rash after being given a course of a form of penicillin called ampicillin. Twenty years later would I still be allergic to penicillin if I were given it now?
A: It's difficult to say. Ampicillin had a particular problem with rashes, particularly in people with glandular fever, so you may not be allergic to other forms of penicillin, such as penicillin

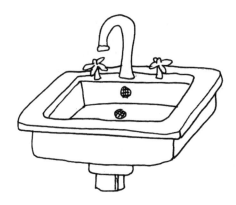

V or amoxicillin. However, it's always best to err on the side of caution, so I wouldn't prescribe any form of penicillin for you. There are other non-penicillin antibiotics that would probably do the same job for you in any infection and would not put you at risk of a severe reaction.

Q: Why do doctors no longer take any notice of the colour of the tongue? I remember as a child the doctor always looking at my tongue to check that I was healthy. Now my doctor says that it's not important. My tongue is always covered with a soft white fur. It isn't painful. What can it be? Should I try to scrape it off?

A: Tongue examination was thought to be important in Victorian times when doctors knew very little about the true causes of disease. They thought its appearance reflected what was going on inside the person. Now we may look at the tongue for any local signs of infection of the tongue, but not to check general health. There are better ways of doing that. However, the white fur may be a fungal or bacterial infection. Your doctor may well be able to give you something for it.

Q: I've noticed that my husband tends to drop off to sleep in the passenger seat when I'm driving the car, even during the day. He gets plenty of sleep through the night, though his snoring does disturb me. Is this anything to worry about? He tells me that it's a compliment to my driving that he is relaxed enough to fall asleep.

A: I'm sure he is right on that last point, but I'm unhappy about the combination of daytime sleepiness and night-time snoring. That sounds like sleep apnoea until proven otherwise, and you need to deal with it. Is he overweight? Is his collar size above 16, for example? If so, ask him to visit his doctor, who will want to know more about his sleep habits, and may even refer him to the local sleep laboratory. He or she will also check on his cardiovascular health, as sleep apnoea is a 'red flag' symptom for potential heart disease. In the meantime, if your husband is carrying excess weight, get him to lose it. That could solve both the drowsiness and the snoring, and it may prevent a possibly lethal heart arrhythmia, the risk of which is raised in people with sleep apnoea.

Q: My son has an abscess at the root of a tooth. It is very painful, but the dentist will only give an antibiotic and not remove the tooth until after it is healed. Meanwhile he is in a lot of pain. Why won't he take the tooth out?

A: Your dentist is quite right. The aim is to get the infection to die down before he treats the tooth. Then he may be able to save the tooth. To try to remove it while it is infected risks complications, like spreading the infection into the bloodstream, to cause septicaemia. It is much safer to use an antibiotic first. Your son should take adequate amounts of painkillers in the meantime.

Q: I have sciatica. My doctor won't ask for an X-ray, but instead has given me exercises to do. Shouldn't he make sure that there isn't a disc out of place?

A: Frankly, no. Less than 5 per cent of all cases of sciatica are linked to disc problems, and even then the treatment would be the same whether there was one or not. The vast majority of sciatica cases are caused by back muscle strains that eventually heal themselves, and they heal faster with active exercises. Your doctor's initial examination of your back would have confirmed that you have this form of sciatica. So he is right not to waste resources on X-rays and to get you straight on to the correct treatment.

Q: I'm 69, smoke a pipe and rarely drink. I have pains in my heels at night that make me get out of bed and stamp around. Painkillers haven't helped. Can you suggest something to relieve this pain?

A: Pain in the heels at night suggests a circulation problem in your legs that needs to be checked. Your doctor will feel for your pulses in your legs (in the groin, behind your knees, at your ankle and in your foot) to see if there is a blockage. If there is, you will need investigations. In the meantime, stop the smoking: the nicotine in your blood may well be the problem. It powerfully narrows the arteries in your legs. Do see your doctor.

Q: I've lost two stones recently, and my doctor has found that I'm anaemic. I've been sent for a bowel endoscopy. Why is that? I've always had normal bowel movements, and have never passed blood.

A: I'm afraid I must be blunt. Your doctor is following the guidelines for early diagnosis of bowel cancer. Seventeen per cent of men and women who are found to have what is called iron deficiency anaemia on routine testing turn out to have bowel cancer, even though they have not had any symptoms (like diarrhoea or bleeding) or signs (like lumps in the abdomen). So your doctor is trying to rule out cancer as a cause for the anaemia. Anaemia isn't an illness in itself – it is a sign that there is an underlying problem that has to be found and cured. You may have been leaking tiny amounts of blood every day in your motions – enough to make you anaemic, but not enough to show.

Q: My husband has low back pain, and says that we should lie on a very hard mattress. I feel much more comfortable on one that will 'give' a little. Do I really have to change our mattress for his sake? I don't have back pain.

A: The hard mattress story was put in doubt in the early 2000s by a really well-conducted trial of types of mattress for back pain sufferers. It showed that over 90 days, people with back pain did better sleeping on 'medium firm' than on 'very firm' mattresses. So you don't have to sleep on a hard bed – a reasonably firm one will do. You need a little 'give' that will help the mattress mould around your shape. Patients with chronic back pain tell me that memory foam mattresses or mattresses topped by a memory foam cover have helped them to sleep. I hope that doesn't upset your husband.

Q: My mother died from bowel cancer at the age of 45. I'm now 22 and have been told I have hundreds of polyps in my bowel. The surgeon recommends I have my colon removed now, before I develop cancer. I attend for regular follow-up. Do I really have to have my colon removed, or can I wait until something turns up at the follow-up clinic, maybe years from now? I really don't want the operation.

A: Sadly, your surgeon is probably right in his advice. You have a very high chance of developing cancer in one of these polyps, and sometimes even with close follow-up the change to cancer can be so fast that it can spread too far between the clinic appointments. Do ask for a long appointment with your consultant and your doctor, and if necessary for a second opinion, so that you are absolutely clear about your particular risk. Each person is different. But your consultant has probably the experience of hundreds of cases behind him – and that matters a lot when the decision has to be made. Remember that when your colon is removed your chance of developing cancer drops from near 100 per cent to zero. That's quite a consideration.

Q: I am frankly depressed. I'm not bad enough to do myself harm, but can't see a future ahead in which I could be happy. I don't want to take antidepressant drugs. Are there alternatives?

A: Your doctor will want to talk to you at length about your mood and how to help you. That isn't just about prescribing drugs, but counselling about your feelings, attitudes and emotions and how to respond to them in a way that can lift you, rather than make you feel worse. You may be recommended to have cognitive behaviour therapy at your local clinic. However, antidepressants will help you as well. The two approaches of counselling and behaviour therapy and drugs can help a lot.

Don't despair – do get help. You shouldn't try to work through this alone.

Q: I have developed Bell's palsy. One side of my face is twisted and I dribble saliva from the corner of my mouth. I've had it for a month now. What are the chances of my recovering completely?

A: Very high. More than 90 per cent of people with Bell's palsy start to recover in a few months, and recover completely in the long term. You may have to be patient, however. It can take six months or more before you are happy with your face again.

Q: I had lumbar disc surgery for severe sciatica four months ago. The pain down the back of my legs has gone, but I still have pain in my shins especially when walking. Will this go away in time?

A: It may not without further tests and treatment. Pain in the front of the leg comes from a different disc, so that the operation would not have helped it. Tell your doctor that you still have this pain.

Q: I have an underactive thyroid for which I take thyroxine. I am now told that I have a high cholesterol level. Could the thyroxine have raised my cholesterol level?

A: No. Low thyroid function and a high cholesterol often go together. If anything, by giving you more energy and making you more active, thyroxine should drive your cholesterol down. However, improving your thyroid function won't necessarily correct your cholesterol level, so you may need treatment, such as a statin drug along with thyroxine, for both.

Q: Is it true that there are drugs to improve your intellect? A friend says that some prescription amphetamines can do this. What's the catch?

A: In 2008 there was a report in *Nature* about people who had bought drugs like this online. The two commonest were methylphenidate, licensed for the treatment of attention-deficit hyperactivity in children, and modafinil, mainly used to reduce narcolepsy (excessive sleepiness) and also (off licence) to help shift-workers keep awake at the right times. The problem is that all the trials, naturally, have been in people with the disorders for which they have been licensed. We don't know what they will really do, long term, to normally healthy people. They are amphetamines, after all, so they lead to addiction, and they carry an impressive list of side effects, including tremor, loss of coordination, dry mouth and eyes, appetite changes, indigestion, abdominal pains, palpitations, anxiety, sleep problems, and a host of symptoms related to overactivation of the nervous system. They can even cause psychosis and mania. There's no real evidence that they improve intellect: they may help you to think faster, but not more effectively. I definitely wouldn't take them myself.

Q: I've been very anxious lately, because I can't get a job, and often have pains in my chest. I'm 21. When I told my doctor about the chest pains I was frankly insulted when he asked if I had been using crack cocaine. I'm not a drug abuser: why did he have to ask that?

A: Because using crack cocaine causes chest pains in older teenagers and young adults, especially in people who seem over-anxious. The doctor had to rule it out. Be happy that your doctor had the knowledge and experience to be aware of this possibility and could ask about it. If your doctor can't ask straight questions because he might shock you, then you don't have a good relationship with him.

Q: A friend has had two fits recently and was told by his doctor he must not drive. I know he is still driving. He says that he only had the fits at night, when he wasn't driving, so he should be safe. Is he right?

A: If this is a new case of epilepsy he must not drive until he has been fully assessed by the appropriate specialist. His doctor would have asked him to inform the DVLA about his convulsions, and that he was under investigation. He could have a fit behind the wheel, and that would obviously be a danger to himself and other people around him. You should make sure that he contacts the DVLA. If he continues to drive you have no alternative but to tell the appropriate people yourself.

Q: What causes restless legs? I have this urge to keep moving my legs at night in bed. Is there a treatment?

A: We don't know the cause. It affects women more than men, and is particularly severe in pregnancy in the last three months. Pills aren't usually the answer. Keeping cool in bed, avoiding caffeine-containing drinks for several hours before bedtime, and relaxing in a warm bath before going to bed can help. Some drugs, like diuretics, given for heart failure and high blood pressure, antidepressants and anti-epilepsy drugs have been implicated in causing restless legs, and are best taken in the mornings rather than in the evenings. Once your legs start twitching, walk about, stretch your leg muscles and have another bath. If after all this they are still a serious problem, then 'dopamine receptor agonist' drugs (prescription names include bromocriptine, pergolide, pramipexole and ropinirole) have been reported to be of some use. However, they all have side effects, so before you take them you need to talk to your doctor about them. And expect your doctor to refer you for a neurological examination, too, to rule out any underlying problem in your nervous system.

Q: My father and my great-uncle developed dementia in their sixties. I'm in my late thirties and have a son aged eight. Can we do anything to prevent us developing it? Do those brain-training systems on computers work?

A: First, you and your son are not at a significantly higher risk of developing dementia than is the general population. Very few cases of dementia are inherited. Most are related to lifestyle and environment. For example, there is evidence that early dementia is linked to alcohol and tobacco misuse, past head injuries, physical inactivity, depression and type 2 diabetes linked to obesity. So the best advice is to keep a healthy lifestyle. Most important seems to be to keep up a good level of exercise. Recently, studies showed that learning a musical instrument when a child, and especially becoming a professional musician, lays down extra connections between the brain cells that should protect people from developing dementia. Other possible ways to improve brain connections, as yet unconfirmed but showing real promise, is to eat plenty of blueberries and to bask in a bright light for two hours a day! Sadly, the biggest study of brain training (in 11,000 volunteers and organized by the Medical Research Council Unit in Cambridge) didn't show any improvement in their subjects' intellect.

Index

vaccines 75
vitamin D 17

warfarin 12
wax 55

.